ABC of
Diabetes

Sixth Edition

ABC series

An outstanding collection of resources - written by specialists for non-specialists

The *ABC series* contains a wealth of indispensable resources for GPs, GP registrars, junior doctors, doctors in training and all those in primary care

- **Now fully revised and updated**

- **Highly illustrated, informative and practical source of knowledge**

- **An easy-to-use resource, covering the symptoms, investigations, treatment and management of conditions presenting in your day-to-day practice and patient support**

- **Full colour photographs and illustrations aid diagnosis and patient understanding of a condition**

For more information on all books in the *ABC series*, including links to further information, references and links to the latest official guidelines, please visit:

www.abcbookseries.com

Diabetes

Sixth Edition

Tim Holt

Health Sciences Research Institute, Warwick Medical School, University of Warwick, Coventry, UK

Sudhesh Kumar

Clinical Sciences Research Institute, Warwick Medical School, University of Warwick; *and* WISDEM, University Hospital, Coventry, UK

WILEY-BLACKWELL

A John Wiley & Sons, Ltd., Publication

BMJ|Books

This edition first published 2010, © 2010 by Tim Holt and Sudhesh Kumar
Previous editions: 1983, 1988, 1993, 1998, 2003

BMJ Books is an imprint of BMJ Publishing Group Limited, used under licence by Blackwell Publishing which was acquired by John Wiley & Sons in February 2007. Blackwell's publishing programme has been merged with Wiley's global Scientific, Technical and Medical business to form Wiley-Blackwell.

Registered office: John Wiley & Sons Ltd, The Atrium, Southern Gate, Chichester, West Sussex, PO19 8SQ, UK

Editorial offices: 9600 Garsington Road, Oxford, OX4 2DQ, UK
    The Atrium, Southern Gate, Chichester, West Sussex, PO19 8SQ, UK
    111 River Street, Hoboken, NJ 07030-5774, USA

For details of our global editorial offices, for customer services and for information about how to apply for permission to reuse the copyright material in this book please see our website at www.wiley.com/wiley-blackwell

Library of Congress Cataloging-in-Publication Data

Holt, Tim A.
  ABC of diabetes. – 6th ed. / by Tim Holt and Sudhesh Kumar.
    p. ; cm.
  Rev. ed. of: ABC of diabetes / Peter J. Watkins. 5th ed. 2003.
  Includes bibliographical references and index.
  ISBN 978-1-4051-7784-9
  1. Diabetes – Popular works. I. Kumar, Sudhesh. II. Watkins, Peter J. ABC of diabetes. III. Title.
  [DNLM: 1. Diabetes Mellitus. WK 810 H758b 2010]
  RC660.4.H65 2010
  616.4′62 – dc22

                                                                2009013393

ISBN: 978-1-4051-7784-9

A catalogue record for this book is available from the British Library

Set in 9.25/12 Minion by Laserwords Private Limited, Chennai, India
Printed and bound in Malaysia by KHL Printing Co Sdn Bhd

1   2010

Contents

Foreword

The prevalence of diabetes has exploded over the past two decades. In 2000 there were an estimated 151 million people with diabetes worldwide. The latest estimates for 2010 are 285 million, with a conservative estimate that this number will rise to 438 million over the next 20 years. By far the majority of these are people with type 2 diabetes but the numbers with type 1 diabetes are also rising. This is placing an ever increasing burden on health services and, obviously, prevention at the population level is vital. But the needs of the individual with diabetes are also of paramount importance. Good care is vital to slow down and prevent the development of both microvascular and macrovascular complications. This is crucial both for the individual and for the long-term costs of care.

One result of this increase is that it has become obvious that care of people with diabetes is the responsibility of all parts of the health-care system with the biggest impact on primary care – both medical and other professionals. Systematic care is vital – and complex algorithms are not the answer. Education is also vital and needs to be targeted, particularly at primary care workers.

The present text fits the bill admirably. It is targeted at primary care practitioners and nurses. It could be called the A to Z of diabetes rather than the ABC! It goes systematically through all stages of diabetes – from diagnosis to a lucid discussion of the complications as well as providing a useful guide to the organisation of diabetes care in general practice. It should also be an obligatory text for medical students who receive woefully little diabetes teaching. Overall, this book fills a yawning gap and should have a place in every general practice and on every diabetes nurse practitioner's shelves.

Professor Sir George Alberti
Senior Investigator, Imperial College, London
Emeritus Professor of Medicine,
University of Newcastle upon Tyne

Preface

Building on the established reputation of the ABC of Diabetes series, this completely rewritten sixth edition contributes insights and materials from the Diabetes educational programme of Warwick Medical School. Originating in a primary care context, the Warwick teaching programme draws equally on secondary care expertise based at the Warwickshire Institute for Diabetes, Endocrinology and Metabolism (WISDEM), hosted by University Hospital, Coventry. The wider metabolic context in which diabetes occurs is an important research interest at Warwick and this will hopefully be reflected through the pages of this book.

New technologies create opportunities for diagnostic, therapeutic and organisational innovation. The development of an increasingly integrated software environment through the UK National Health Service provides means of organising and monitoring diabetes care that were not available to previous generations of health professionals. This book explains how organisational infrastructure is as important as any other aspect in ensuring high quality diabetes care. Whilst using UK examples to illustrate these principles, we hope that readers in other countries may recognise this common need. The interaction between primary and secondary care, including criteria for cross-referral is of central importance in developing services based on locally available resources.

The book promotes the patient-centred approach throughout. It responds to the increasing importance of the primary care setting, whilst also covering the hospital management of emergencies. People living with diabetes in the twenty-first century generally expect to be involved in treatment decisions, if not to lead them, but they equally expect their health care professionals to be well informed and to provide authoritative guidance, particularly when things don't go to plan. We hope that the insights offered by this book will equip practitioners for both circumstances – managing the routine 'surveillance' scenarios when risk factor control and quality of life issues are the priorities, whilst retaining the ability to respond to acute situations of metabolic instability or fulminating complications.

These are exciting times, as new discoveries and technologies are making significant improvements in outcomes for people with diabetes. Thus, new developments in diabetes care can easily overtake current policy. We have attempted to incorporate all recent developments, for example, the diagnostic criteria for diabetes, as discussed in the first chapter. Whilst we would advise readers to keep a watchful eye on new developments, we feel confident that this book will provide a sound understanding of the guiding principles of diabetes management.

Tim Holt
Sudhesh Kumar

Acknowledgements

This book would not have been possible without the generous support and advice of colleagues at Warwick Medical School and the University Hospital, Coventry. A number are involved as tutors on the Warwick Diabetes courses and are also practising clinicians, both in primary and secondary care, ensuring that this book reflects contemporary UK practice.

We are indebted to numerous individuals who have generously provided figures, tables, photographs and offered suggestions during proof-reading. We are particularly grateful to colleagues who helped with the preparation of the book including: Dr Aresh Anwar (Consultant Physician), Dr Paul O'Hare (Clinical Reader in Medicine), Dr Sailesh Sankar (Consultant Physician), Dr Vinod Patel (Clinical Reader in Medicine), Dr Ponnusamy Saravanan (Associate Clinical Professor in Diabetes), Mr Gurdev Deogan (Senior Podiatrist, University Hospital, Coventry), Dr Noreen Kumar (Foundation Year House Officer, St James's Hospital, Leeds), and Mr Gary Misson (Consultant Ophthalmologist, Warwick Hospital).

Others who have provided advice and educational resources include Dr Roger Gadsby (Senior Clinical Lecturer, Warwick Medical School), Wendy Goodwin (Diabetes Specialist Nurse, University Hospital, Coventry), and Claire Holt (Practice Nurse, Kenyon Medical Centres, Coventry).

We are also very grateful to Professor Andrew Boulton (Professor of Medicine, University of Manchester), Professor Cliff Bailey (Professor of Pharmacology, Aston University) and Dr Cathy Lloyd (Open University) for their helpful comments and suggestions on improving the manuscript.

Finally, we thank Mrs Susan Watson for help with preparation of the manuscript, and the publishing team at Wiley-Blackwell for their support and advice at all stages.

T.H.
S.K.

CHAPTER 1

Diagnosing Diabetes

Tim Holt[1] and Sudhesh Kumar[2]

[1]Health Sciences Research Institute, Warwick Medical School, University of Warwick, Coventry, UK
[2]Clinical Sciences Research Institute, Warwick Medical School, University of Warwick; and WISDEM, University Hospital, Coventry, UK

OVERVIEW

- Diabetes produces a variety of clinical presentations, from acute to gradual onset
- Currently, the diagnosis should be based on two separate tests unless the patient is clearly symptomatic in which case only one positive test is required
- New World Health Organization diagnostic criteria based on glycosylated haemoglobin are expected in the near future
- A combination of genetic and environmental factors contribute to the risk of diabetes
- Impaired glucose regulation is an important risk factor both for future diabetes and cardiovascular disease
- Distinction between random and fasting samples is essential in interpreting the significance of borderline blood glucose levels
- Impaired glucose tolerance can only be diagnosed by oral glucose tolerance test

---

Introduction

Diabetes mellitus is a common metabolic disorder that is defined by chronic hyperglycaemia. Besides symptoms related to hyperglycaemia itself such as thirst, polyuria and weight loss, it may also cause potentially life-threatening acute hyperglycaemic emergencies. It is a major cause of morbidity and premature mortality from long-term complications such as cardiovascular disease, blindness, renal failure, amputations and stroke. With good control of hyperglycaemia established early on and continued life-long, an individual with diabetes can enjoy a good quality of life and reduce the risk of these long-term complications that are so detrimental to their life and wellbeing.

Prevalence of diabetes

In the United Kingdom we have an estimated 1.8 million people with diabetes. However, based on screening studies it is believed that up to a million more may be undiagnosed (see pages 15 and 17).

ABC of Diabetes, 6th edition. By T. Holt and S. Kumar.
Published 2010 by Blackwell Publishing.

The prevalences of both type 1 and type 2 diabetes are increasing. Type 2 diabetes is increasing far more rapidly, driven by increasing life expectancy and the epidemic of obesity. It is believed that there will be as many as 300 million people with diabetes worldwide by the year 2025. Most of this increase will occur in developing countries. The majority of children have insulin-requiring type 1 diabetes, whilst the vast majority of those aged >25 years will have type 2 diabetes (Figure 1.1).

Types of diabetes

The types of diabetes have been classified by the WHO. Type 1 diabetes (previously referred to as insulin-dependent diabetes mellitus or IDDM) is due to absolute insulin deficiency and is usually an autoimmune disease leading to the destruction of the insulin-secreting beta cells in the pancreas. In some cases the cause of destruction of the beta cells is not known.

Type 2 (previously known as non-insulin dependent diabetes mellitus or NIDDM) results from relative insulin deficiency that may be associated with varying degrees of insulin action defects known collectively as insulin resistance.

For a practising clinician the implication of this diagnosis is that patients with type 1 diabetes require insulin straight away and insulin should not be stopped as it is life-preserving. Type 2 patients can progress through several stages and may require insulin later on in their disease.

Risk factors for diabetes

Genetics. Genetic susceptibility is important for both types of diabetes. Family history of type 1 diabetes or other autoimmune diseases such as autoimmune thyroid disease is associated with a higher risk of developing type 1 diabetes in the family. Inheritance in type 2 diabetes is far more complex as there are many underlying causes. Furthermore, the risk varies according to the particular sub-type of type 2 diabetes. A family history of type 2 diabetes in a first degree relative is a strong risk factor for diabetes in that individual.

Obesity. Apart from family history, obesity is a very important risk factor for diabetes. For a given degree of obesity, central or 'apple-shaped' obesity is associated with a much higher risk of

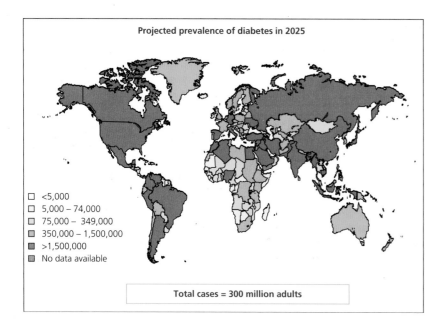

Projected prevalence of diabetes in 2025

☐ <5,000
☐ 5,000 – 74,000
☐ 75,000 – 349,000
▨ 350,000 – 1,500,000
■ >1,500,000
▨ No data available

Total cases = 300 million adults

Figure 1.1 Projected prevalence of diabetes in 2025. Reproduced with permission from the World Health Organisation. The World Health Report. Life in the 21st Century: a vision for all. Geneva: WHO, 1998.

progression to type 2 diabetes than those who have lower body obesity or are 'pear-shaped'. Those with a body mass index (BMI) of >25 k/m² or high waist circumference (Table 1.1) are at a higher risk of developing diabetes and should be encouraged to take regular exercise and eat healthily (Figure 1.2).

Age. Beta cell function declines with age, indeed if we live long enough all of us have the potential to develop diabetes at some stage. With an aging population an increase in prevalence of diabetes can be expected.

Ethnicity. People of South Asian or Afro-Caribbean origin are at higher risk of developing diabetes. They are also more likely to have type 2 diabetes presenting at a young age and usually have poorer risk factor control. South Asian patients have a high risk of developing diabetic renal disease and also coronary artery disease. Afro-Caribbean patients are more likely to have strokes and have

a higher risk of gestational diabetes. South Asian and Hispanic children may develop type 2 diabetes.

Initial presentation and diagnosis

The commonest presentation is tiredness, thirst, polyuria, weight loss, pruritus vulvae or balanitis. It is not uncommon for this

Table 1.1 The International Classification of adult underweight, overweight and obesity according to BMI (adapted from WHO guidelines, http://apps.who.int/bmi/index.jsp?introPage=intro_3.html)

Classification	BMI(kg/m²)	
	Principal cut-off points	Additional cut-off points
Underweight	<18.50	<18.50
Normal range	18.50–24.99	18.50–22.99
		23.00–24.99
Overweight	≥25.00	≥25.00
Pre-obese	25.00–29.99	25.00–27.49
		27.50–29.99
Obese	≥30.00	≥30.00
Obese class I	30.00–34.99	30.00–32.49
		32.50–34.99
Obese class II	35.00–39.99	35.00–37.49
		37.50–39.99
Obese class III	≥40.00	≥40.00

Source: Adapted from (WHO 1995, 2000, 2004).

Figure 1.2 'Apple'-shaped fat distribution (central obesity with intra-abdominal adiposity) carries a higher cardiovascular and diabetes risk than 'pear'-shaped fat distribution.

diagnosis to be missed for years, and a significant proportion of those with type 2 diabetes remain undiagnosed. Insidious symptoms mean that the patients generally tend to ignore them. This is one reason why complications are often seen at diagnosis in patients with type 2 diabetes. A number of cases with type 2 diabetes are now diagnosed at insurance examinations or through opportunistic testing when the patient has presented for some other problem to the general practice or hospital.

The diagnosis of diabetes must not be taken lightly by a clinician as the consequences for the individual are significant and life-long. For those presenting with severe symptoms, evidence of long-term complications or severe hyperglycaemia at presentation, the diagnosis is quite straightforward and can be made using only one diagnostic blood glucose measurement. In asymptomatic individuals presenting with mild hyperglycaemia, the diagnosis should only be established on the basis of at least two abnormal test results. In future, the recently published recommendation is that HbA1c values will be used rather than plasma glucose as it has been in the past (Box 1.1).

Box 1.1 Recommendation of the International Expert Committee

For the diagnosis of diabetes:

- The HbA1c assay is an accurate, precise measure of chronic glycaemic levels and correlates well with the risk of diabetes complications.
- The HbA1c assay has several advantages over laboratory measures of glucose.
- Diabetes should be diagnosed when HbA1c is ≥6.5%. Diagnosis should be confirmed with a repeat HbA1c test. Confirmation is not required in symptomatic subjects with plasma glucose levels ≥11.1 mmol/l.
- If HbA1c testing is not possible, previously recommended diagnostic methods (e.g. FPG or 2 hour OGTT, with confirmation) are acceptable.
- HbA1c testing is indicated in children in whom diabetes is suspected but the classic symptoms and a casual plasma glucose ≥11.1 mmol/l are not found.

For the identification of those at high risk for diabetes:

- The risk for diabetes based on levels of glycemia is a continuum; therefore, there is no lower glycemic threshold at which risk clearly begins.
- The categorical clinical states pre-diabetes, IFG, and IGT fail to capture the continuum of risk and will be phased out of use as HbA1c measurements replace glucose measurements.
- Those with HbA1c levels below the threshold for diabetes but ≥6.0% should receive demonstrably effective preventive interventions. Those with HbA1c below this range may still be at risk and, depending on the presence of other diabetes risk factors, may also benefit from prevention efforts.

(Adapted from: The International Expert Committee. International Expert Committee Report on the role of the HbA1c assay in the diagnosis of diabetes. *Diabetes Care* 2009;32:1327–34; 2009)

Glucose tolerance test

A glucose tolerance test should be performed in the morning after an overnight fast. It is important that the patient should have had a normal diet for the preceding 3 days and should not restrict carbohydrate intake drastically. The test should also not be performed during an acute illness or following prolonged bedrest. Plasma glucose concentrations are measured fasting and then 2 hours after a drink of 75 g of glucose in 250–350 ml of water (in children: 1.75 g/kg up to maximum of 75 g). Several proprietary preparations are available and these are often flavoured to make items palatable. Table 1.2 shows normal values and interpretation of abnormal values during an oral glucose tolerance test (OGTT). The role of oral glucose tolerance tests is set to change given the recent recommendations over the use of HbA1c as a preferred means of diagnosing diabetes (Box 1.1).

Interpretation of the oral glucose tolerance test results

Impaired fasting glycaemia (IGF)
Fasting glucose between 6.1 and 6.9 mmol/l in the absence of abnormal values after the glucose load is defined as impaired fasting glycaemia. Conversion to diabetes is not invariable but it is important to reassess once a year, and in future this is likely to be through HbA1c measurement (see Box 1.1). Individuals with IFG should be advised about a healthy life-style and to avoid obesity.

Impaired glucose tolerance (IGT)
Once again conversion to diabetes is not invariable and patients may either persist with impaired glucose tolerance, revert to normal glucose tolerance or progress to type 2 diabetes. Obese individuals should be advised to try and lose weight through diet and exercise. The implications of this diagnosis for pregnancy are different and this is considered further in Chapter 17.

IGF and IGT are collectively known as *impaired glucose regulation* but these terms may become outdated as HbA1c becomes the recommended means of diagnosing diabetes and identifying those at risk (see Box 1.1).

Diabetes mellitus
A fasting glucose of greater than or equal to 7.0 mmol/l or a 2-hour glucose value of greater than or equal to 11.1 mmol/l suggests

Table 1.2 WHO criteria for the diagnosis of diabetes mellitus based on venous plasma samples.

	Fasting (mmol/l)	2-hour sample following oral glucose challenge (mmol/l) in OGTT
Normal	<6.1	<7.8
Impaired fasting glycaemia (IFG)	6.1–6.9	<7.8
Impaired glucose tolerance (IGT)	<7.0	7.8–11.0
Diabetes mellitus	≥7.0	≥11.1

Table 1.3 Conversion of DCCT aligned HbA1c measurements to the new IFCC standard.

HbA1c	
DCCT aligned (%)	IFCC (mmol/mol)
4	20
5	31
6	42
6.5	48
7	53
7.5	59
8	64
9	75
10	86
11	97
12	108

diabetes, but in future this will be based on HbA1c (Box 1.1). The glucose tolerance test does not indicate the type of diabetes, this is usually determined on the basis of other presenting features and is discussed further below. Young age at presentation (especially less than 17 years), presence of other autoimmune endocrine diseases (such as hypothyroidism, pernicious anaemia, Addison's disease, vitiligo) in the patient or family members, or significant weight loss are features that suggest type 1 diabetes.

Diabetes in children

Abnormal blood glucose readings in a child or adolescent up to the age of 17 years should be taken seriously as they may have type 1 diabetes and it is important to avoid delay in treatment, especially when they present with very high blood glucose levels. In those with mild hyperglycaemia or where there is doubt, HbA1c should be measured (see Box 1.1).

New units for reporting HbA1c (glycosylated haemoglobin)

Diagnosing diabetes has in the past been based on blood glucose values, but this is likely to change in the near future to a definition based on glycosylated haemoglobin (HbA1c). The measurement of HbA1c has required standardisation of reporting across the world. Table 1.3 gives a chart for converting the older DCCT aligned units (%) to the new International Federation of Clinical Chemistry (IFCC) units (mmol/mol).

Identifying patients in need of insulin or urgent referral to hospital

Insulin is life-saving in those with type 1 diabetes and is also indicated in all patients with marked hyperglycaemia or significant weight loss particularly if ketosis is detected in the urine or blood. Children are much more likely to have type 1 diabetes. Any form of hyperglycaemia in pregnancy is also an indication for insulin. Patients who fail to achieve adequate glycaemic control on oral agents should also be given insulin. A patient who is unable to eat and drink normally and has marked hyperglycaemia due to a concomitant illness will require insulin and may need to be seen in hospital urgently.

Metabolic syndrome

Type 2 diabetes, hypertension, dyslipidaemia and central obesity often present in the same individual. This clustering of chronic risk factors has been called the metabolic syndrome. Therefore, the presence of central obesity, hypertension or dyslipidaemia should prompt the clinician to look for diabetes. It should be noted that the majority of patients with metabolic syndrome do not yet have overt type 2 diabetes but may have either undiagnosed diabetes or impaired glucose tolerance. It is here that the concept of metabolic syndrome is particularly useful. As patients with diabetes should have other cardiovascular risk factors treated intensively anyway, identifying metabolic syndrome in such patients may not alter management.

Delaying the onset of type 2 diabetes

In those identified as being 'at risk', life-style changes to increase physical activity and a diet with modest calorie restriction, less saturated fat and more dietary fibre can significantly reduce the rate at which impaired glucose tolerance progresses to type 2 diabetes. It has been demonstrated that even older people can successfully undertake the life-style programmes required. This is discussed in more detail in Chapter 4.

Further reading

DECODE Study Group. Is the current definition for diabetes relevant to mortality risk from all causes and cardiovascular and non-cardiovascular diseases? *Diabetes Care* 2003;**26**:688–96.

Freemantle N, Holmes J, Hockey A, Kumar S. How strong is the association between abdominal obesity and the incidence of type 2 diabetes? *Int J Clin Pract* 2008;**62**:1391–6.

The International Expert Committee. International Expert Committee Report on the role of the HbA1c assay in the diagnosis of diabetes. *Diabetes Care* 2009;**32**:1327–34.

World Health Organization. *Definition, Diagnosis and Classification of Diabetes Mellitus and its Complications: Report of a WHO Consultation.* World Health Organization, Geneva, 1999. WHO/NCD/NCS 99.2

CHAPTER 2

Types of Diabetes

Tim Holt[1] and Sudhesh Kumar[2]

[1]Health Sciences Research Institute, Warwick Medical School, University of Warwick, Coventry, UK
[2]Clinical Sciences Research Institute, Warwick Medical School, University of Warwick; and WISDEM, University Hospital, Coventry, UK

> **OVERVIEW**
>
> - A number of different pathological mechanisms produce chronic hyperglycaemia, the hallmark of clinical diabetes
> - These mechanisms produce different patterns of presentation and therefore different types of diabetes
> - Important pathways include autoimmune destruction of beta cells in type 1 diabetes, and insulin resistance with gradual decline in beta cell function in type 2
> - Diabetes may also result from drug therapy or from systemic disease affecting other organs as well as the pancreas
> - There is increasing interest in the classification of sub-types of diabetes, which is assisting in the personalisation of treatments for affected individuals

Introduction

Diabetes mellitus is not one disease. It is defined as chronic hyperglycaemia that may be caused by one or more of numerous underlying processes. Some of these cause diabetes directly by interfering with beta cell function or through significant defects in insulin action. In other cases diabetes is part of a more general disorder affecting many other organs or systems. Examples include some endocrinopathies, drug- or chemical-induced diabetes; diabetes related to certain infections and diabetes associated with certain genetic syndromes.

Although one might argue that management of diabetes is empirical and that knowledge of the underlying causes does not alter management for most patients, this is changing. For some distinct sub-types of diabetes, there are clinical implications for the patient and their family. In the future, this is likely to lead to increasing personalisation of drug therapy.

Type 1 diabetes

Type 1 diabetes results from destruction of the beta cells in the islet cells of Langerhans in the pancreas (Figure 2.1). This usually results in more or less absolute deficiency of insulin. In most cases,

ABC of Diabetes, 6th edition. By T. Holt and S. Kumar.
Published 2010 by Blackwell Publishing.

this is due to autoimmune destruction of the islets. This results from a combination of genetic susceptibility and poorly understood environmental triggers that initiate the disease process. It is believed that this process starts a long time before the illness actually presents. There is, therefore, an opportunity for prevention of diabetes in the future in this group of patients. Type 1 diabetes is far more common in those with a history of other autoimmune disorders such as coeliac disease, thyroid disease, pernicious anaemia and Addison's disease. If there is a strong family history of any of these disorders, the risk of type 1 diabetes in these families is higher.

Genetic factors predisposing to type 1 diabetes

The strong concordance of type 1 diabetes in monozygotic twins suggests a major role for genetic factors. The major

(a)

(b)

Figure 2.1 Beta cell destruction after 50 years of type 1 diabetes.

histocompatibility complex antigens are thought to be important. Most type 1 patients show either DR3 or DR4, whilst DR2 is thought to be protective against diabetes.

Autoantibodies in type 1 diabetes

Islet cell autoantibodies are present at diagnosis but will gradually decline and disappear in ensuing years. This means that if there is diagnostic uncertainty, islet cell antibodies can be checked early during presentation. Specific tests have been devised recently including anti-GAD (glutamate decarboxylase) antibodies and also anti-IAP (inhibitor of apoptosis protein) antibodies. The presence of both together is associated with a significantly higher risk of developing type 1 diabetes.

The use of these tests in clinical practice is restricted to situations where there is doubt about the diagnosis of the type of diabetes and to distinguish from type 2 diabetes. Clinically, the implication is that if the tests are negative the patient might then not require insulin. Attempts to prevent type 1 diabetes in these susceptible individuals has thus far not proved successful.

Type 2 diabetes

Type 2 diabetes is a complex heterogeneous condition and recent genetic studies have revealed numerous sub-types. Children presenting with mild hyperglycaemia present diagnostic problems as they may have latent slowly progressing type 1 diabetes. These children may then progress to requiring insulin. On the other hand, with increasing prevalence of obesity more children are now presenting with type 2 diabetes, particularly from ethnic minorities. In the USA, in some areas, up to 50% of children with diabetes are now presenting with the type 2 form.

Latent autoimmune diabetes in adults (LADA) is thought to comprise about 5% of all patients with type 2 diabetes. These people have autoantibodies usually seen in type 1 diabetes, but their clinical presentation is like someone with type 2 diabetes. This is a group that may present an excellent opportunity for subsequent prevention of diabetes if an effective intervention can be developed to prevent further beta cell destruction.

Monogenic diabetes (previously referred to as maturity onset diabetes in the young, MODY)

Monogenic diabetes is the term used for a collection of conditions that cause diabetes now shown to result from single gene defects. One feature of these conditions is that they show autosomal dominant inheritance patterns where the disease appears to be vertically transmitted (e.g. through several generations). It is also diagnosed before the age of 25 years, but, unlike type 1 diabetes patients, monogenic diabetes patients do not often require insulin for at least 5 years after diagnosis. Genetic testing in these cases can confirm the particular sub-type of diabetes. This can have significant clinical implications. Patients with HNF1α (hepatocyte nuclear factor 1α) mutations, for example, exhibit exquisite sensitivity to sulphonylureas and can be successfully treated with tablets. Knowledge of the mutation, therefore, can help in the management of this disorder, even in children who would otherwise have been put onto insulin. This is also one form of type 2 diabetes where we would use a sulphonylurea in preference to metformin when initiating therapy. Patients with HNF1β have renal cysts. Patients with glucokinase mutations are less common but the diagnosis is significant for the individual and their families. Such patients are much less likely to develop complications of diabetes because they mainly have mild fasting hyperglycaemia without significant post meal hyperglycaemia.

Maternally inherited diabetes with deafness (MIDD)

This is a form of diabetes due to mutations in mitochondria, most commonly related to 3243A > G mitochondrial DNA mutation. Mitochondria in an individual are inherited from the mother rather than from the father, therefore one clue would be evidence of strong maternal transmission of diabetes, particularly when this is associated with a sensorineural deafness. Some patients may also have peripheral vision problems, particularly night blindness. These patients often require insulin.

(a)

(b)

Figure 2.2 Lipodystrophy affecting the buttocks (a) but not the abdomen (b).

Lipodystrophies

It has been known for a long time that marked defects in adipose tissue distribution may be associated with diabetes. For example, complete absence of subcutaneous adipose tissue as in generalised lipodystrophy or partial lipodystrophies with absence of fat in the face and torso are associated with diabetes and dyslipidaemia. However, more recently a much more common disorder of adipose tissue distribution, familial face-sparing lipodystrophy has been recognised. These patients often have excess fat on the face, neck, abdomen and also visceral fat. They show marked lack of fat in the gluteal area and in the limbs (Figure 2.2). Often patients also have acanthosis nigricans, seen particularly in the axilla or the back of the neck (Figure 2.3). These patients present with an insulin-resistant diabetes, often with hypertriglyceridaemia. Marked hypertriglyceridaemia can be a risk factor for pancreatitis and should be managed with low-fat diet and lipid-lowering medication.

Other insulin-resistant syndromes

Other rarer causes of insulin-resistant syndromes may present in childhood, with failure to thrive, growth problems and also acanthosis nigricans. Paradoxically, these children may exhibit fasting hypoglycaemia and yet once they develop diabetes may require large doses of insulin to control hyperglycemia. If such disorders are suspected, referral to a specialist will be required as the management can be quite difficult.

Figure 2.3 Acanthosis nigricans in the axilla (a) and behind the neck (b).

Further reading

Jafar-Mohammadi B, McCarthy MI. Genetics of type 2 diabetes mellitus and obesity – a review. *Ann Med* 2007;**18**:1–9.

Lindgren CM, McCarthy MI. Mechanisms of disease: genetic insights into the etiology of type 2 diabetes and obesity. *Nat Clin Pract Endocrinol Metab* 2008;**4**:156–63.

Murphy R, Ellard S, Hattersley AT. Clinical implications of a molecular genetic classification of monogenic beta-cell diabetes. *Nat Clin Pract Endocrinol Metab* 2008;**4**:200–13. Epub 2008 Feb 26. Review.

CHAPTER 3

Helping People Live with Diabetes

Tim Holt[1] and Sudhesh Kumar[2]

[1]Health Sciences Research Institute, Warwick Medical School, University of Warwick, Coventry, UK
[2]Clinical Sciences Research Institute, Warwick Medical School, University of Warwick; and WISDEM, University Hospital, Coventry, UK

OVERVIEW

- Patient-centred priority setting and supported self-management form the modern approach to diabetes care
- Control targets should be tailored to the individual
- Patients are more likely to adhere to treatment plans that they have formulated themselves
- Self-efficacy and 'ownership' of the condition should be nurtured through structured education

Introduction

Living with diabetes is a long personal journey. Throughout the journey patients require information, education, support and self-management skills. They also require prescribed medication, monitoring, surveillance and regular review. This journey is a joint venture between the individual, their carers and a multidisciplinary team of health professionals (Box 3.1).

Box 3.1 **Aims of treatment of diabetes**

- Absence of symptoms
- Avoidance of severe hypoglycaemia
- Control of blood glucose to patient-centred targets
- Control of other cardiovascular risk factors
- Prevention, early detection and effective treatment of complications
- Lifestyle sufficiently flexible to suit the person's needs
- Normal life expectancy

Patient-centred priority setting

In the past, patients were expected to passively follow the doctor's instructions. Those who failed to reach targets were simply not complying. This approach was never very effective in diabetes,

but it is increasingly insufficient in the modern world of patient autonomy, access to information, and personal responsibility for health. We now know that individuals are much more likely to adhere to decisions they have formulated themselves. The emphasis of diabetes care should be self-management, supported by a team of health professionals (Figure 3.1).

Shared decision making

The Autonomous Patient: Ending paternalism in medical care by Angela Coulter (2002) suggests three models of clinical decision making (Table 3.1).

The shared decision making model is increasingly used in primary care, where patients are usually not acutely ill. The clinician must provide and share information, whilst the patient

Figure 3.1 Discussing treatment goals.

Table 3.1 Models of clinical decision making.

Professional choice	Shared decision making	Consumer choice
Clinician decides, patient consents	Information shared, both decide together	Clinician informs, patient makes decision

Reproduced with permission from Coulter A, *The Autonomous Patient*, 2002.

ABC of Diabetes, 6th edition. By T. Holt and S. Kumar.
Published 2010 by Blackwell Publishing.

must be prepared to discuss personal values and preferences. Both accept shared responsibility for the treatment decisions. A successful clinician-patient relationship built on mutual trust allows the model to be adapted flexibly to the situation. Development of a serious acute illness might shift the emphasis towards Professional choice, whilst the need to choose a hospital for non-urgent cataract surgery might be purely a Consumer choice.

Targets

Treatment targets are often recommended for the entire population with diabetes, but in fact should be tailored to different patient types depending on co-morbidity, life expectancy, patient preferences and other factors. Discussing personalised goals with the patient and sharing responsibility for keeping within targets is an important step in successful control of risk factors. Generally: aim for HbA1c ≤7.0% (53 mmol/mol) in all patients and ≤6.5% (48 mmol/mol) in the majority; keep blood pressure ≤140/80 for everyone and ≤130/80 if possible; control total serum cholesterol to ≤4.0 mmol/l and LDL cholesterol to ≤2.0 mmol/l. This is particularly important in type 2 patients with established cardiovascular disease or risk factors for it. In practice, this includes the majority with type 2 diabetes (see Chapter 5).

Realistic weight reduction targets should be set. Gradual, sustainable weight loss is far more beneficial than sudden loss, which is initially encouraging but then demoralising when the weight returns. The same applies to physical activity, which should be gradually increased to a moderate level over a period of time.

Some targets are easier to achieve than others (Table 3.2). Controlling blood pressure and lipids is usually possible provided the individual concords with prescribed drug therapy. The more difficult areas are those requiring self-management skills and lifestyle change. Glycaemic targets may need adjusting based on risk of hypoglycaemia, and hypoglycaemia awareness. A frail, elderly patient may have different needs and priorities to a younger, more active individual (Box 3.2).

Table 3.2 Type 2 diabetes – meeting the needs.

Readily achieved	Difficult to achieve
Blood pressure control	Durable control of glycaemia
Lipid management	Post-prandial glucose levels
Screening for complications	Abdominal obesity
Glycaemic control in early stages of disease	Smoking cessation
	Physical inactivity

Box 3.2 Key attributes to nurture in our patients

Knowledge about the condition, and how it may affect them now and in the future
'Ownership' of their diabetes
Shared responsibility for decision making
The confidence to plan changes and take control
Trust in us to act for their benefit

Main issues to cover in the first consultation

- The biochemical basis for diabetes in lay terms (raised blood sugar, insufficient insulin, body not responding to insulin properly)
- Diabetes can cause problems with a number of organs and body systems, which can be prevented through a joint effort between the patient and the practice team
- Controlling blood glucose levels reduces the chances of complications of diabetes, but controlling blood pressure and cholesterol are equally important
- The importance of lifestyle: weight control and exercise not only reduce blood glucose, blood pressure, and cholesterol, but also make the body's own insulin work more effectively
- Realistically, over time there is a tendency for the glucose levels to rise further, so that medication usually needs to be 'stepped up' as time goes by, even in the patient who 'does everything right'. It is important that patients don't feel demoralised by such an escalation (Box 3.3)
- Mention in outline the range of treatments – lifestyle change, tablets, insulin. Discuss insulin in a positive way (even though not needed now) and not as a 'last desperate resort'. This will help in future if the time comes when it is needed
- Refer to 'lifestyle' or 'dietary' changes rather than to 'dieting' to avoid the patient believing that their treatment will involve a strict 'crash' diet that they are unlikely to sustain

Box 3.3 Lifestyle changes and drug therapy

Lifestyle change is important for the majority of patients, but some may feel disinclined to change their behaviour if they are immediately prescribed drug therapy. A period of behavioural adaptation following diagnosis before drugs are commenced may be beneficial unless the indication is strong. Three months is the traditional interval

Keeping on the same side

Newly diagnosed patients sometimes feel overwhelmed at the prospect of self-managing a complex and potentially serious medical condition. Such individuals need structured education, support and confidence building, provided by a consistent and integrated team of health professionals. Developing our patients' knowledge and skills towards a state of self-efficacy (Box 3.4) is one of the most valuable things we can offer them in the early stages of diabetes.

Box 3.4 Self-efficacy

'Self-efficacy' is a key element to the success of behavioural change in diabetes. The term refers to the individual's personal ability to take action and make changes. Self-efficacy is the basis for a number of diabetes management interventions, including DAFNE, DESMOND and the Diabetes Manual

Figure 3.2 Armande Voizin, played by Judi Dench. From the film *Chocolat*. Photo credit: David Appleby/Courtesy of Miramax Film Corp.

Armande, the character played by Judi Dench in the 2000 film *Chocolat*, conceals her insulin-dependent diabetes at the local chocolaterie. Defying pressure from her daughter to enter institutional care, she follows the village's general slide into temptation, and dies through overindulgence in chocolate. Set in rural France in 1959, the story reflects the shifting social trend towards freedom of choice, and her death is portrayed as a victory for personal autonomy. But the basis for her defiance is a lack of self-efficacy, and the absence of a non-judgemental clinician she can trust. Adult patients rarely opt for the rebellion route if given sufficient support and a feeling of ownership of their condition.

How can we help patients change their lifestyles?

- Engage with the patient from the time of diagnosis
- Be clearly 'on the same side'
- Reinforce positive moves to change and praise achievements, even small ones
- Give consistent, supportive messages from all members of the team, using written material
- Encourage the patient to access educational resources themselves, including reliable websites that support the same messages as the health team
- Take it a little at a time and set realistic short-term goals
- Emphasise the need to *maintain* change, which is more difficult than achieving it in the first place
- Provide the actual figures: most patients can easily understand the basic indices and targets and by feeling a sense of 'ownership' of the data will accept responsibility for them (Box 3.5)

Structured education

As well as regular input from the practice team, patients may benefit from entering a structured education programme. This is particularly valuable following diagnosis but can be offered at any time. In the UK, available programmes include DESMOND and The Diabetes Manual (for type 2 patients) and DAFNE for type 1 patients.

DESMOND (Diabetes Education and Self-Management for Ongoing and Newly Diagnosed) is an educational package to help people with type 2 diabetes, particularly those who are newly diagnosed. It has been shown to have benefits on weight loss and smoking cessation and positive improvements in beliefs about illness. All aspects of self-management are covered, in a group setting.

The Diabetes Manual is also designed for type 2 patients but involves one to one education and is therefore suitable for those who prefer to avoid group education settings. In addition to a comprehensive manual, audiotapes are provided, and practice nurses are trained to deliver the educational material.

DAFNE (Dose Adjustment For Normal Eating) is a 5-day training programme for people with type 1 diabetes. It involves learning accurate carbohydrate counting and adjustment of insulin doses according to need. It is suitable for well-motivated patients whose diabetes is less than adequately controlled, who have been diagnosed for at least 6 months, and who are prepared to monitor four to six times a day and inject frequently using a basal bolus regimen. It is based on the idea that tailoring insulin doses to the person's usual diet (which is in principle unrestricted) is the best way of achieving glycaemic control without increased hypoglycaemia. It has been shown in a randomised controlled trial to improve HbA1c levels (as well as quality of life scores) without increasing the frequency of severe hypoglycaemia.

'Yo-yoing'

There is a thriving market for faddish diets and alternative dietary advice, which should be resisted. Patients are understandably attracted to media publicity or anecdotal accounts of rapid weight loss, but such approaches are rarely sustainable, and 'yo-yoing' (fluctuating weight with no overall trend towards reduction) has been shown to be actively harmful. Yo-yoing is less likely if newly diagnosed patients are presented with a positive image of healthy food rather than a simple list of prohibited items. Many type 2 patients have developed diabetes at least partly because they adore food. To disregard this long-established devotion is simply futile.

Their interest in food needs to be redirected rather than extinguished. Offering a wide range of healthy options in a positive way will avoid the impression of a gastronomic prison sentence. See Chapter 10 for dietary advice for diabetes.

Semantics

Whilst many do not object to the term 'diabetic', a proportion finds it stigmatising. The term, when referring to an individual, has been 'banned' from many of the major publications including the *British Medical Journal*. Its use as an adjective (e.g. 'the diabetic foot') is generally considered acceptable, but it should no longer be used as a noun. The same has occurred for people with epilepsy. The term 'patient' is appropriate in context, but we should not forget that for most of the time people with diabetes are not ill.

Summary

Modern diabetes care needs to be patient-centred, recognising that people are on the whole more likely to succeed in achieving targets if they themselves have formulated, or helped formulate, the management plan. Care should also be individually tailored, whilst maintaining standards that are common to all patients. Confidence building to promote self-efficacy, and keeping on the same side, are important and deserve the necessary time commitment particularly in the early stages after the diagnosis.

Further reading

Coulter A. *The Autonomous Patient: Ending paternalism in medical care. The Nuffield Trust*. The Stationary Office, London, 2002.

DAFNE Study Group. Training in flexible, intensive insulin management to enable dietary freedom in people with type 1 diabetes: dose adjustment for normal eating (DAFNE) randomised controlled trial. *BMJ* 2002; **325**:746

Davies MJ, Heller S, Skinner TC, *et al*. Diabetes Education and Self Management for Ongoing and Newly Diagnosed Collaborative. Effectiveness of the diabetes education and self management for ongoing and newly diagnosed (DESMOND) programme for people with newly diagnosed type 2 diabetes: cluster randomised controlled trial. *BMJ* 2008;**336**(7642):491–5.

Sturt J, Taylor H, Docherty A, *et al*. A psychological approach to providing self-management education for people with type 2 diabetes: the Diabetes Manual. *BMC Fam Pract* 2006;**7**:70.

Department of Health. *The expert patient: a new approach to chronic disease management for the twenty-first century*. London: Department of Health, 2001; www.ohn.gov.uk/ohn/people/expert.

Tattersall R. The expert patient: A new approach to chronic disease management for the twenty-first century. *Clin Med JRCPL* 2002;**2**:227–9.

CHAPTER 4

Early Detection and Prevention of Diabetes

Tim Holt[1] and Sudhesh Kumar[2]

[1]Health Sciences Research Institute, Warwick Medical School, University of Warwick, Coventry, UK
[2]Clinical Sciences Research Institute, Warwick Medical School, University of Warwick; and WISDEM, University Hospital, Coventry, UK

OVERVIEW

- Hyperglycaemia is among the top five determinants of worldwide mortality
- Increasing life expectancy is the main driver of the global diabetes 'epidemic'
- Increasing obesity and physical inactivity add to this effect producing rising prevalence of type 2 diabetes in younger people
- Prevention and early detection of diabetes are essential to offset the associated morbidity and mortality
- Diabetes may be prevented by lifestyle interventions
- Those at risk of type 2 diabetes are also at risk of cardiovascular disease and represent a large population with unmet health needs

---

Introduction

Two hundred and fifty million people worldwide have diabetes, and 80% of these are likely to die of cardiovascular disease. The escalating prevalence is often referred to as an 'epidemic', but unlike an infectious disease, which typically burns itself out after a time, there is no suggestion that this will happen to the global diabetes problem. Figure 4.1 shows the projected increase in estimated numbers of people with diabetes in different regions of the world by 2030, and the trend by age band in developed and developing countries.

Changes in population demography

Expansion of the over-65 population, occurring most rapidly in developing countries, is the single most important factor driving this trend, and rising obesity prevalence will only add to these estimates. Established market economies currently have the highest prevalence, but countries experiencing industrialisation are likely to witness the greatest increase in patient numbers and in many of these areas health care provision is under-developed.

ABC of Diabetes, 6th edition. By T. Holt and S. Kumar.
Published 2010 by Blackwell Publishing.

Type 2 diabetes in the young

Meanwhile, in developed countries a different phenomenon is occurring – the increasing recognition of type 2 diabetes in adolescents and young adults. This rise is largely linked to obesity. In the USA, this problem disproportionately affects African-American and Hispanic populations (Cali and Caprio 2008) (Figure 4.2).

Increasing obesity prevalence, particularly in industrialised nations, results largely from behavioural rather than genetic factors. High calorie foods containing simple carbohydrate and saturated fat, together with increasingly sedentary lifestyle patterns, have fuelled this trend. This problem must be addressed at all levels – individual choice, clinician advice and public health measures – in order to influence the food industry.

Impacting on the diabetes epidemic

Improved nutrition, environmental conditions and medical care, all extending life-expectancy to age bands where diabetes is more prevalent, are driving the epidemic. The solution must come through early detection and intervention through preventive measures. This means not only reducing progression to diabetes, but also targeting groups at risk of diabetes for multifactorial cardiovascular risk reduction.

Pre-diabetes and macrovascular disease

Microvascular complications of diabetes are related to duration and severity of raised blood glucose. There is a much weaker relationship between hyperglycaemia and the macrovascular complications, which may have been brewing for years before the onset of diabetes itself. Macrovascular disease is associated with insulin resistance, which may predate beta cell insufficiency and overt hyperglycaemia by decades, but is typically accompanied by hypertension and dyslipidaemia. This has raised interest in this early phase, and the concept of 'pre-diabetes', as much of the morbidity associated with it is preventable. Beta cell function itself declines progressively prior to the diagnosis of diabetes (Figure 4.3).

The annual worldwide mortality associated with 'higher than optimal blood glucose levels' (which includes diabetes and the less severe borderline states) may be three times higher than that of

Figure 4.1 Projected numbers of people (thousands) with diabetes from 2000 to 2030 by region, and overall global rise in prevalence by age band. Reproduced with permission from Wild S, Roglic G, Green A *et al. Diabetes Care* 2004;**27**:1047–1053.

Figure 4.2 Childhood obesity is increasing the prevalence of type 2 diabetes in young people.

Figure 4.3 Beta cell function in the natural history of T2DM – data from UKPDS. Reproduced with permission from Holman R. *Diabetes Res Clin Pract* 1998;**40**(Suppl. 1):S21–S25.

Table 4.1 Relative risk of ischaemic heart disease and stroke for 1 mmol/l increase in fasting plasma glucose, by age group (after adjustment for confounding and regression dilution bias). Reproduced with permission from Danaei G, Lawes CMM, Vander Hoorn S, *et al. Lancet* 2006;**368**:1651–9.

	<60 years	60–69 years	≥70 years
Ischaemic heart disease	1.424	1.196	1.196
Stroke	1.360	1.284	1.081

diabetes itself (Danaei *et al.* 2006). The cardiovascular risk rises with increasing glycaemia from a level well below the threshold used to diagnose diabetes (Table 4.1). This puts raised blood glucose, whether or not high enough to be called diabetes, among the five top determinants of worldwide mortality, accounting for 3.16 million deaths a year (Diabetes Prevention Program Research Group 2002) (Figure 4.4).

The tip of the iceberg

In industrialised societies, and increasingly in the developing world, for every person in the community with diabetes there are many with the metabolic syndrome (Box 4.1) or other forms of 'pre-diabetes'. A quarter of the world's adults are estimated to have the metabolic syndrome as defined by the International Diabetes Federation

(see Box 4.2). Such people have a 20% risk of developing diabetes. Whilst many are currently living in the economically developed nations, less industrialised countries are developing similar lifestyle patterns and catching up (Table 4.2).

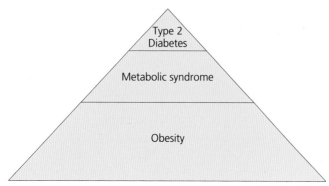

Figure 4.4 The 'iceberg' of preventable cardiovascular risk.

Box 4.1 **The metabolic syndrome**

Type 2 diabetes is a complex metabolic disorder, lying at one end of a spectrum of progressively impaired glucose regulation, insulin resistance, and beta cell insufficiency. Central obesity, hypertension and dyslipidaemia usually accompany this constellation and together represent the 'metabolic syndrome'. Identifying this condition gives us an opportunity to delay the onset of diabetes and control the other cardiovascular risk factors that are part of the syndrome

Box 4.2 **The metabolic syndrome: International Diabetes Federation definition**

Central obesity (see Table 4.2) plus any two of the following four factors:

Raised Triglyceride level: ≥1.7 mmol/l, or specific treatment for this lipid abnormality
Reduced HDL cholesterol: <40 mg/dl (1.03 mmol/l*) in males and <50 mg/dl (1.29 mmol/l*) in females, or specific treatment for this lipid abnormality
Raised blood pressure: systolic BP ≥130 or diastolic BP ≥85 mm Hg, or treatment of previously diagnosed hypertension
Raised fasting plasma glucose ≥5.6 mmol/l, or previously diagnosed type 2 diabetes

*If above 5.6 mmol/l, an oral glucose tolerance test is strongly recommended but is not necessary to define the presence of the syndrome

Silent damage

Type 2 diabetes tends to develop gradually over long periods of time. Complications may be established, or even advanced, at the time of diagnosis. These affected up to 50% of newly diagnosed type 2 patients in the UKPDS Study. Macrovascular complications may precipitate awareness of a previously unrecognised diagnosis. An individual may present with an acute myocardial infarction or stroke, and be diagnosed with diabetes during his/her first admission to hospital. Alternatively, the patient may very gradually develop symptoms of thirst and polyuria. Established complications such as retinopathy or albuminuria may have progressed silently over the preceding years.

Should we screen the population for diabetes?

The early phase of diabetes in which people are asymptomatic but nevertheless developing serious and preventable complications would argue strongly in favour of a screening programme. But whilst there are a number of identifiable factors that raise an individual's risk, most of them (such as age and body mass index) are very non-specific, so that a screening programme would need to involve a large proportion of the adult population. A further issue is the choice of screening test. Random blood glucose levels are relatively non-specific, leading to large numbers requiring follow-up depending on the threshold used. Fasting levels are more specific but may miss people whose abnormal glucose regulation affects their response to carbohydrate challenge rather than their fasting levels. This is more likely to apply to South Asian people. Such individuals will only be identified by an oral glucose tolerance test (OGTT). The OGTT is considered the 'gold standard' but is not always reproducible. Patients with impaired glucose tolerance can only be identified using OGTT.

Screening for raised cardiovascular risk

The overlap between type 2 diabetes, impaired glucose regulation and raised cardiovascular risk has, in the UK, resulted in a shift away from diabetes screening, and towards individualised cardiovascular risk assessments. This is intended for those without either established vascular disease or diabetes in the over-40 age group. These

Table 4.2 Ethnicity specific definition of central obesity.

Country/Ethnic group	Waist circumference	
Europids	Male	≥94 cm
In the USA, the ATP III values (102 cm male; 88 cm female) are likely to continue to be used for clinical purposes	Female	≥80 cm
South Asians, Chinese and Japanese	Male	≥90 cm
Based on a Chinese, Malay and Asian Indian population	Female	≥80 cm
Ethnic South and Central Americans	Use South Asian recommendations until more specific data are available	
Sub-Saharan Africans	Use European data until more specific data are available	
Eastern Mediterranean and Middle East (Arab) populations	Use European data until more specific data are available	

If BMI is >30 kg/m^2, central obesity can be assumed and waist circumference does not need to be measured.
Adapted from: International Diabetes Federation ethnicity-specific definitions of central obesity.

assessments include a random blood glucose estimation followed by further investigation of borderline or raised levels. They also involve the use of cardiovascular risk algorithms using the known risk factors, together with other relevant information such as ethnicity, family history, body mass index, waist circumference and random plasma glucose (followed if necessary by fasting plasma glucose or OGTT). This serves as a screening programme for vascular risk factors including diabetes and impaired glucose regulation.

Preventing diabetes in those at risk

Can we delay the onset of diabetes, or prevent it altogether?

The opportunity to reduce cardiovascular risk in individuals with 'pre-diabetes' is one benefit of identifying impaired glucose regulation. Another is the opportunity to delay or prevent progression to diabetes itself. The Diabetes Prevention Programme in the USA (Diabetes Prevention Programme Research Group 2002), and the Finnish Diabetes Prevention Study (Tuomilehto *et al.* 2001) both found a 58% reduction in the risk of developing diabetes when such people were treated with lifestyle interventions including nutritional management, weight loss and exercise (see Figure 4.5). More recently, a study has demonstrated the relationship between adherence to a 'Mediterranean' diet and reduced risk of future diabetes (Martínez-González, de la Fuente-Arrillaga and Nunez-Cordoba 2008). The case for drug therapy is more controversial.

Preventing diabetes – lifestyle management or drug therapy?

Drug therapy to prevent diabetes seems an attractive option. Whilst concordance is always an issue, prescribed drug therapy may be adhered to more effectively than lifestyle changes for many individuals. A number of agents have been shown to be effective, summarised in a systematic review by Gillies and colleagues (Gillies *et al.* 2007). These include metformin, rosiglitazone, acarbose and orlistat. However, a concern is that the drug therapies may be simply masking the onset of diabetes. There are also practical issues. If we offer a person drug therapy for this reason, at what point do we retest them for diabetes, and do we withdraw the drug before the test? Unless this policy is very clearly understood, there is a risk that people with impaired glucose regulation may end up with partially treated, undiagnosed diabetes, masked by drug therapy. The diabetes is then not monitored adequately, because the person has never achieved the diagnostic criteria for diabetes and is not on the diabetes register. The importance of the diabetes register as a means of organising diabetes care is emphasised in Chapter 18.

Whilst trials of behavioural interventions have demonstrated reduced risk of diabetes and cardiovascular disease, there are difficulties in translating these benefits into clinical practice. Even in the more controlled context of a clinical trial involving patients who already have a diagnosis of diabetes, maintaining lifestyle change is not easy. Figure 6.3 in Chapter 6 gives the success rates in the UKPDS study. The Steno-2 study of a multifactorial intervention was similarly affected by fairly low rates of ideal target achievement, particularly for glycaemia and systolic blood pressure (Figure 4.7). Despite this, both studies demonstrated clear benefits for the intervention group.

The 'missing population' with diabetes

Undiagnosed diabetes in the UK

In addition to those who are known to have diabetes, currently amounting to around 3.5% of the UK population, an estimated

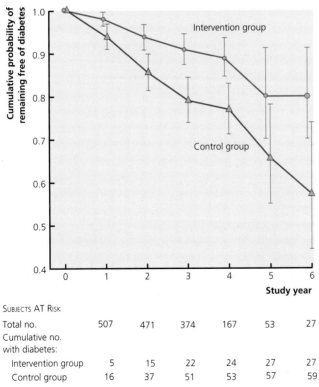

Subjects at Risk						
	0	1	2	3	4	5	6
Total no.	507	471	374	167	53	27
Cumulative no. with diabetes:						
Intervention group	5	15	22	24	27	27
Control group	16	37	51	53	57	59

Figure 4.5 Improved risk of developing diabetes in the Finnish Diabetes Prevention Study, which involved a lifestyle intervention. Reproduced with permission from Tuomilehto J, Lindström J, Eriksson JG, *et al. N Engl J Med* 2001;**344**:1343–50.

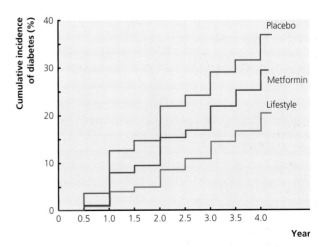

Figure 4.6 Reduction in risk of developing diabetes in the United States Diabetes Prevention Program. The lifestyle intervention reduced the risk by 58% and was significantly more effective than metformin. Reproduced with permission from Tuomilehto J, *et al. N Engl J Med* 2001;**344**:1343–50.

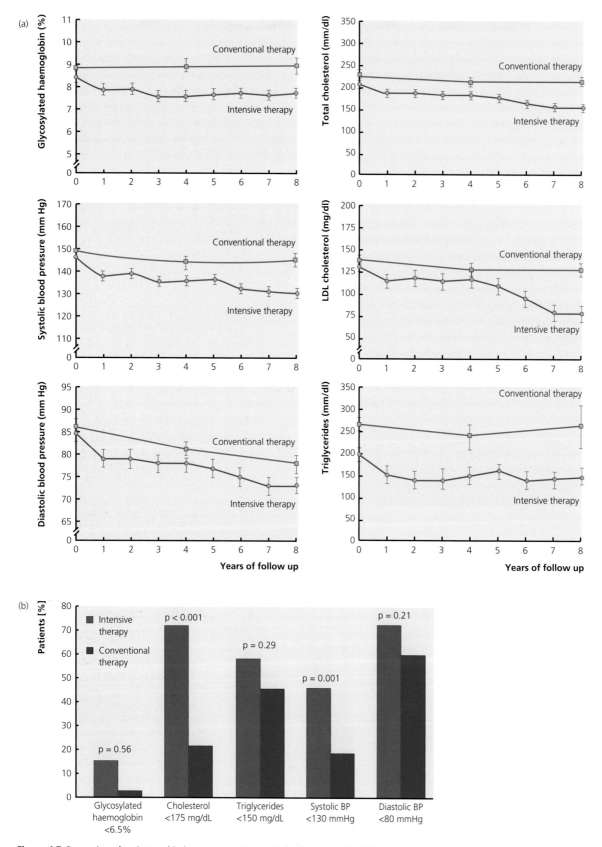

Figure 4.7 Proportion of patients achieving treatment targets in the Steno-2 study. (a) Demonstrates significant differences in risk factor levels between the two trial arms. However (b) highlights the difficulties in achieving ideal targets, even during a well organised research trial. Adapted from Gæde and colleagues (2003).

1% have diabetes that is either undiagnosed or unrecorded on diabetes registers. Six hundred thousand people are failing to receive structured care and follow-up for a serious chronic condition, even in a country with a highly developed health care infrastructure. Other estimates put the figure closer to a million. Adding still further to this problem, large numbers with borderline blood glucose levels are unidentified and likely to suffer highly preventable cardiovascular events. It is this group that are particularly likely to benefit from interventions to prevent diabetes and macrovascular disease.

Raising awareness

Much publicity has been aimed towards the general public to improve early diagnosis of diabetes. This involves two strategies (Box 4.3). Firstly, people should be made aware of the symptoms of diabetes, so that they report them to their health professionals; and secondly, patients in high-risk groups based on ethnicity, family history or other factors should be made aware of arrangements for case finding through regular testing.

> Box 4.3 **Cornerstones of early diabetes detection**
>
> - Raised awareness of the importance of early detection among the general public and health professionals
> - Low threshold for investigating potential diabetes symptoms
> - Effective follow-up of borderline blood glucose levels (see Box 4.4)
> - Active case finding in high-risk groups
> - Regular surveillance in selected patients

Case finding for diabetes

Active measures to detect the 'missing population' with type 2 diabetes include patient awareness raising, e.g. posters encouraging the public to report symptoms of thirst or polyuria, or to be tested if a family history or other risk factors are present. Health professionals can ensure that people at risk of undiagnosed diabetes are invited for testing (Box 4.4). This includes the following groups:

- Those with features of the metabolic syndrome, see Box 4.1
- Those with established cardiovascular disease or hypertension, who should have a blood glucose test in some form done every 3 years. Any random value 6.1 mmol/l or higher should be followed up with a fasting test and/or HbA1c
- Those with a family history of type 2 diabetes, particularly in a first-degree relative
- Ethnic groups, e.g. South Asian, Afro-Caribbean, Hispanic, Pacific Islander

Investigation of suspicious symptoms

The diagnosis of diabetes is often missed simply because the condition is not considered as a diagnostic possibility when the individual reports symptoms. Particular settings when this may occur include:

- Failure to include blood glucose measurement in the assessment of tiredness, weight loss or urinary symptoms

- Investigation of urinary symptoms using a midstream specimen of urine (MSU) that excludes infection but does not include urinalysis for glucose
- An assumption that the patient's symptoms are due to prostatic disease, urinary infection, or bladder instability

This problem often affects type 2 patients whose symptoms develop gradually and are frequently attributed to ageing. But an alarming number of type 1 patients are also diagnosed late, and are then at risk of life-threatening ketoacidosis.

> Box 4.4 **Using primary care databases to identify undiagnosed diabetes**
>
> A study published in 2008 Holt *et al.* demonstrated the use of routinely collected general practice data to identify patients at risk of undiagnosed diabetes. The investigators simply looked for raised blood glucose readings in primary care electronic health records. Out of 3.6 million records examined, 0.1% of patients had no diagnosis of diabetes and a random blood glucose level at the most recent measurement ≥11.1 mmol/l, or a fasting level ≥7.0 mmol/l. This computer search was termed 'Strategy A'. When projected to the UK population this would amount to 60,000 individuals. A further Strategy 'B' used a lower threshold of 7.0 mmol/l (random or fasting) for the most recent reading, and identified 0.9% of the survey population, projecting to 528,000 individuals nationwide. Some of these people will have had the reading taken recently and be in the usual process of follow up. But in over a third of the 'A' patients and half of the 'B' patients, the last recorded value was more than 1 year ago. Some of these people may belong to the missing population with diabetes. As a result of this study, computer software was designed and installed in the majority of UK practices to assist practitioners in identifying them.
>
> **Time since last blood glucose measurement**
>
>
>
> Proportion of blood glucose measurements identified by strategies A and B according to time interval since the measurement.

Summary

Type 2 diabetes develops gradually and produces non-specific symptoms, so is often diagnosed late. There is a large missing population with undiagnosed diabetes, and an even larger population with the 'metabolic syndrome', at risk of both diabetes and cardiovascular disease. Opportunities are missed to reduce cardiovascular risk in such patients, whose typically raised body mass index, waist circumference, hypertension and hyperlipidaemia should make them easy to recognise in health care settings. Active programmes of weight reduction, nutritional management and physical activity are proven to reduce progression to diabetes in those at risk, and should be widely promoted. Early detection and intervention are the only means through which the epidemic of diabetes and associated cardiovascular disease can be curtailed. It is among the most important health care challenges of our time.

Further reading

Cali AMG, Caprio S. Prediabetes and type 2 diabetes in youth: an emerging epidemic disease? *Curr Opin Endocrinol, Diabetes Obesity* 2008;**15**: 123–7.

Danaei G, Lawes CMM, Vander Hoorn S, *et al.* Global and regional mortality from ischaemic heart disease and stroke attributable to higher-than-optimum blood glucose concentration: comparative risk assessment. *Lancet* 2006;**368**:1651–9.

Diabetes Prevention Program Research Group. Reduction in the incidence of type 2 diabetes with lifestyle intervention or metformin. *New Engl J Med* 2002;**346**:393–403.

Gæde P, Vedel P, Larsen N, *et al.* Multifactorial intervention and cardiovascular disease in patients with type 2 diabetes. *N Engl J Med* 2003;**348**: 383–93.

Gillies CL, Abrams KR, Lambert PC, *et al.* Pharmacological and lifestyle interventions to prevent or delay type 2 diabetes in people with impaired glucose tolerance: systematic review and meta-analysis. *BMJ* 2007;**334**: 299.

Holman R. Assessing the potential for α-glucosidase inhibitors in prediabetic states. *Diab Res Clin Pract* 1998; **40**(Suppl 1): S21–5.

Holt TA, Stables D, Hippisley-Cox J, *et al.* Identifying undiagnosed diabetes: cross-sectional survey of 3.6 million patients' electronic records. *Br J Gen Practice* 2008;**58**:192–6.

Martínez-González MÁ, de la Fuente-Arrillaga C, Nunez-Cordoba JM. Adherence to Mediterranean diet and risk of developing diabetes: prospective cohort study. *BMJ* 2008;**336**:1348–51.

Tuomilehto J, Lindström J, Eriksson JG, *et al.* Prevention of type 2 diabetes mellitus by changes in lifestyle among subjects with impaired glucose tolerance. *N Engl J Med* 2001;**344**:1343–50.

Wild S, Roglic G, Green A, *et al.* Global Prevalence of Diabetes: Estimates for the year 2000 and projections for 2030. *Diabetes Care* 2004;**27**: 1047–53.

CHAPTER 5

Cardiovascular Disease

Tim Holt[1], Sudhesh Kumar[2], Ponnusamy Saravanan[3] and Vinod Patel[4]

[1]Health Sciences Research Institute, Warwick Medical School, University of Warwick, Coventry, UK
[2]Clinical Sciences Research Institute, Warwick Medical School, University of Warwick; and WISDEM, University Hospital, Coventry, UK
[3]Clinical Sciences Research Institute, Warwick Medical School, Coventry, UK and George Eliot Hospital, Nuneaton, UK
[4]Institute of Clinical Education, Warwick Medical School, Coventry, UK and George Eliot Hospital, Nuneaton, UK

OVERVIEW

- Macrovascular disease including myocardial infarction and stroke is the prime cause of excess mortality in diabetes
- Microvascular disease produces disabling complications including retinopathy and nephropathy
- Vascular outcomes are improved through multifactorial interventions
- Tight control of glycaemia, blood pressure and serum cholesterol usually requires a combination of life-style change and several different drug therapies
- Angiotensin converting enzyme inhibitors are the drugs of first choice for hypertension in people with diabetes unless they are of Afro-Caribbean descent or where there is a possibility of pregnancy
- Almost all patients with type 2 diabetes justify lipid-lowering therapy

---

Introduction

Most people with type 2 diabetes will ultimately die from cardiovascular disease, and many of these prematurely. Vascular complications are highly preventable provided good quality care is maintained consistently throughout the individual's life. Life expectancy is reduced in people with diabetes (Figures 5.1–5.3) for a number of reasons. Preventable cardiovascular disease is the major one. Effective control of cardiovascular risk requires a multifactorial approach (Box 5.1) as described in this chapter.

Box 5.1 Microvascular and macrovascular disease

Tight glycaemic control is particularly effective at reducing microvascular complications (retinopathy, nephropathy, neuropathy), whilst macrovascular disease affecting the larger vessels is more influenced by lipids, blood pressure, body fat distribution and exercise. Blood pressure control (and smoking cessation) has a highly beneficial effect on both micro- and macrovascular disease. So a multifactorial approach addressing all of these factors is extremely important.

ABC of Diabetes, 6th edition. By T. Holt and S. Kumar.
Published 2010 by Blackwell Publishing.

'Buying in' to polypharmacy

In many areas of medicine, polypharmacy is rightly seen in a negative light. With increasing drugs in the regimen, interactions become more common. Patient adherence may be problematic, particularly on divided dose regimens, with the risk of accidental over-dosing. Reactions to medication may occur that are difficult to attribute to a single component of the schedule. All of these problems are more common in the elderly, and particularly in the visually impaired, who may need supervision from a carer and dosette boxes or other aids. However, in diabetes, a multifactorial approach will inevitably require multiple drug therapies. This is not always particularly acceptable to patients, who sometimes feel that the risks of polypharmacy cannot possibly be outweighed. So how do we manage expectations and facilitate the introduction of what is likely for most patients to be a regimen of at least three different drugs?

Explain *at the outset* why polypharmacy in diabetes is worth the potential difficulties. Mention the probable need for multiple therapies before the patient actually needs them. The addition of a second or third antihypertensive may then be accepted as a norm and not seen as a simple 'failure' of monotherapy. The number of different drugs available now make it likely that a suitable combination will be found for the individual. The commonly used

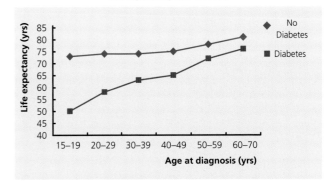

Life expectancy and diabetes

Figure 5.1 Life expectancy is reduced in diabetes, particularly for the young type 1 patients diagnosed in childhood. This Figure is based on a mortality study reported in the 1970s (Goodkin G. *Journal of Occupational Medicine* 1975;**17**(11):716–21). Modern proactive prevention programmes with tight risk factor control and early intervention for emerging complications are changing this pattern.

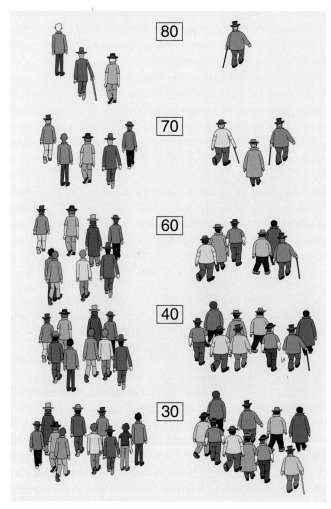

Figure 5.2 How 10 obese men and 10 lean men fare on the journey through life (Joslin, 1941).

drugs are safe for the majority. Controlling blood pressure using two or more different agents is more likely to be successful than using higher doses of single drugs, and less likely to give the side effects that are often associated with the higher rather than middle range doses. The same principle applies to other areas, including glycaemic control, where for instance metformin may be increased from a moderate dose to the maximum licensed dose with little improvement in blood glucose levels but significantly greater risk of abdominal side effects. For hypertension, effective control may be achieved if more than one pathway is blocked, preventing the system from escaping the effects of a single pathway approach. Explaining these principles to the patient may begin to put the concept of polypharmacy in a more positive light.

Blood glucose control

Blood glucose control is particularly important for the prevention of microvascular complications, including retinopathy, nephropathy, and peripheral and autonomic neuropathies. Table 5.1 shows the impact found in a number of studies.

Glycaemic control has a less substantial but still important impact on macrovascular disease (Figure 5.4). The intensive

Table 5.1 Impact of reducing HbA1c on diabetes complications in a number of studies.

Study name	DCCT	UKPDS	Kumamoto	Steno-2
HbA1c	↓2%	↓0.9%	↓2%	↓1.0%
Retinopathy	↓63%	↓17–21%	↓69%	↓58%
Nephropathy	↓54%	↓24–33%	↓70%	↓61%
Autonomic neuropathy	↓60%	–	–	↓63%
CVD	↓41%	↓16%	–	↓53%

Reductions in HbA1c and corresponding reductions in microvascular and macrovascular complications described in major studies of people with type 1 and type 2 diabetes.

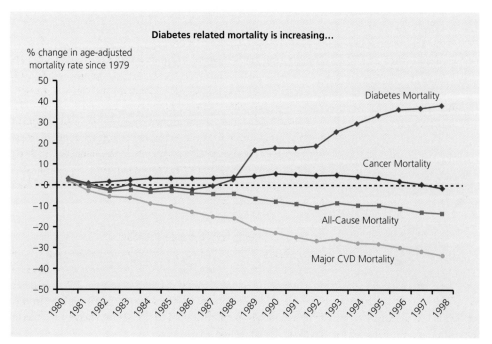

Figure 5.3 Whilst overall cardiovascular mortality is declining, its rate in the population with diabetes is increasing (based on US data). Reproduced from Sobel *et al. Circulation* 2003;**107**; 636–642

Figure 5.4 (a) Glycaemic control improves microvascular outcomes. (b) Blood pressure control reduces risk of both macro- and microvascular complications. Reproduced from Irene M Stratton, Amanda I Adler, H Andrew W Neil. *BMJ* 2000;**321**:405–12 with permission from the BMJ Publishing Group Ltd.

treatment group in the UKPDS study showed 16% fewer myocardial infarctions (Figure 5.5). This study also demonstrated that metformin therapy provided additional CVD benefit over and above the glucose-lowering effect, and therefore should be initiated in all type 2 patients along with the life-style advice. In the STOP-NIDDM trial of patients with impaired glucose tolerance, acarbose significantly reduced the number of CVD events, suggesting that control of post-prandial hyperglycaemia may be beneficial. However, this needs to be proved in prospective studies.

Initial management of blood glucose depends largely on the type of diabetes and the presenting clinical picture. A specific guide is provided in Chapter 6 for type 2 patients.

Tight glycaemic control in older patients–balancing risks and benefits

Increasing numbers of type 2 patients are commencing insulin in order to achieve tight glycaemic control. Benefits of reduced HbA1c need to be balanced against the disadvantages, including the risk of hypoglycaemia. Severe hypoglycaemia may require hospital admission and has a detrimental impact on quality of life. The intensive glucose lowering arm of the ACCORD study was recently halted due to an excess of deaths in those aiming for HbA1c of 6% (42 mmol/mol) or less, although the cause of

these deaths was not simply hypoglycaemia. These findings have triggered a debate about the priority given to tight rather than simply adequate glycaemic control in type 2 diabetes, where it could be argued the major issue is macrovascular disease, unless microvascular complications are established.

Blood pressure control

Antihypertensive medication will be required in the majority of type 2 patients to achieve a target of <140/80 mmHg. This should be complemented with life-style advice to increase exercise and reduce weight and salt and alcohol consumption if appropriate.

Choice of initial antihypertensive therapy

Patients with diabetes whose blood pressure is not within the 140/80 target should be offered antihypertensive drug therapy. First line choice should be an angiotensin converting enzyme (ACE) inhibitor unless the person is of Afro-Caribbean descent, or if there is a possibility of pregnancy. In such cases a calcium channel blocker is appropriate. If the target is still not achieved, a calcium channel blocker or diuretic should then be offered. All three drugs may be given if successful control is still not achieved.

Renal impairment and albuminuria

Microalbuminuria and proteinuria

A positive finding of microalbumin should be confirmed on a second sample and if this is negative a third sample should be checked. An MSU should be sent to exclude infection. Once confirmed, the patient should be treated with an ACE inhibitor or A2RB (sartan) if tolerated, even if their blood pressure is normal, and tighter targets for blood pressure (130/80 mmHg or lower) and HbA1c (aim for 6.5%) should be set, tailored to the individual. Patients with diabetes and hypertension who have dipstick positive **proteinuria** (not just microalbuminuria) usually have widespread vascular disease and are at high risk of cardiovascular events.

Monitoring renal function

Patients with diabetes are at higher risk of renal impairment, particularly older patients who also have hypertension, or those with any degree of proteinuria or microalbuminuria. All patients with diabetes should have estimated glomerular filtration rate (e-GFR) measured at least annually, and many will require more frequent testing. Estimated GFR is a more satisfactory marker of renal function than creatinine alone. Patients with established diabetic nephropathy will require further assessment through 24-hour urinary protein excretion and measurement of actual (rather than estimated) GFR (see also Chapter 12).

Starting ACE inhibitors or A2RBs

Renal function should always be measured before and within 2 weeks after starting a test dose of ACE inhibitor or A2RB, before an increase in dosage is considered. Estimated GFR is a more adequate measure of renal function than creatinine alone in this situation. Ideally, patients should also have this checked after each substantial dose increase.

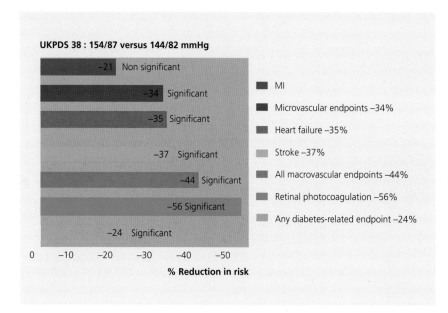

UKPDS 38 : 154/87 versus 144/82 mmHg

- -21 Non significant
- -34 Significant
- -35 Significant
- -37 Significant
- -44 Significant
- -56 Significant
- -24 Significant

■ MI
■ Microvascular endpoints −34%
■ Heart failure −35%
■ Stroke −37%
■ All macrovascular endpoints −44%
■ Retinal photocoagulation −56%
■ Any diabetes-related endpoint −24%

% Reduction in risk

Figure 5.5 Reductions in outcomes attributable to reduced blood pressure in UKPDS. Reproduced from UK Prospective Diabetes Study (UKPDS) Group. *BMJ* 1998;**317**:703–13 with permission from the BMJ Publishing Group Ltd.

Lipid lowering in people with diabetes

Most people with diabetes, particularly those with type 2 diabetes over 40 years, should be considered at risk of cardiovascular disease (Box 5.2). Some are at higher risk than others, and lower risk patients should have their risk reassessed annually (see Box 5.3).

Box 5.2 **The CARDS Study**

The CARDS Study demonstrated a reduction of major cardiovascular events of 37% in people with type 2 diabetes with normal LDL cholesterol levels treated with 10 mg of atorvastatin (see Tables 5.2 and 5.3). Stroke risk was reduced by 48%, and the treatment effect was independent of the pre-treatment cholesterol value.

Box 5.3 **NICE guidelines on Diabetes – type 2 (May 2008) – recommendation for cardiovascular risk assessment:**

Consider a person to be at high premature cardiovascular risk for his or her age unless he or she:

- is not overweight, tailoring this with an assessment of body weight associated risk according to ethnic group
- is normotensive (<140/80 mmHg in the absence of antihypertensive therapy)
- does not have microalbuminuria
- does not smoke
- does not have a high-risk lipid profile
- has no history of cardiovascular disease, and
- has no family history of cardiovascular disease

If the person is considered not to be at high cardiovascular risk, estimate cardiovascular risk annually using the UK Prospective Diabetes Study (UKPDS) risk engine.

Targets

Recommended targets for cholesterol lowering in diabetes are:

- Total cholesterol **<4.0** mmol/l
- LDL **<2.0** mmol/l

Note that LDL can only be measured accurately on a fasting sample (like triglycerides), but for most monitoring purposes random total cholesterols are adequate once control is achieved.

Choice of drug

Most people's cholesterol can be controlled using simvastatin, usually starting at 40 mg at night and titrating upwards if needed to reach target. Those not controlled on 80 mg of simvastatin

Table 5.2 CHD prevention trials with statins in diabetes.

Study	Drug	Number of patients	CHD risk red^n non-diabetics	CHD risk red^n diabetes
Primary prevention				
CARDS	Atorvastatin 10 mg	2838		37%*
HPS†	Simvastatin 40 mg	2912	25%‡	26–33%
Secondary prevention				
CARE§	Pravastatin	586	23%	
4S¶	Simvastatin	202	32%	55%
GREACE	Atorvastatin 24 mg	313		59%
4S reanalysis**	Simvastatin	483	32%	42%
HPS	Simvastatin	3051	24%‡	12% NS

CHD endpoints: *CARDS, acute coronary events; †HPS, first major vascular event; §CARE, absolute risk of coronary events; ¶4S major CHD events; **4S reanalysis, major coronary events.
Cohorts: ‡HPS, risk reduction for the entire cohort (non-diabetics and patients with diabetes).
NS, not statistically significant.

could try a stronger statin such as atorvastatin, again titrating upwards.

On commencing statins, patients should be advised to report unexplained myalgia or muscle weakness. Statin-induced myositis is not common but can be a serious problem if the drug is not withdrawn. However, mild muscle aches without evidence of myositis are much commoner and are not necessarily an indication for statin withdrawal.

Fibrates are appropriate drugs for those intolerant of statins, but can also cause myopathy. They can also be used as second line in those not achieving control with statins alone or if fasting triglycerides remain raised above 2.3 mmol/l despite statin therapy. In patients with previous myocardial infarction, omega-3 fatty acids have been shown to reduce CVD and all-cause mortality. They may also be used if hypertriglyceridaemia persists despite fibrate therapy.

Other ways of reducing cardiovascular risk

Smoking cessation

Smoking in a person with diabetes is particularly harmful. It not only increases the already raised risk of macrovascular disease, but it also increases microvascular complications, particularly nephropathy and retinopathy. Patients with diabetes who smoke should be actively targeted for smoking cessation interventions.

Use of low dose aspirin

Current evidence suggests that, despite their raised cardiovascular risk, people with diabetes may not in fact benefit from low dose aspirin as previous guidelines suggested, and further research is under way to clarify this issue.

Anti-obesity drugs

There is increasing interest in the pharmacological treatment of obesity, but this approach should be part of a structured programme of monitoring and follow-up if it is to be effective. Licensed preparations available in the UK include orlistat and sibutramine. Obesity drugs are discussed further on pages 94–96.

Exercise

Exercise and physical activity are important means of reducing cardiovascular risk and are discussed on pages 45–46. Without regular exercise, attempts to lose weight are much less likely to succeed. Any amount of physical activity is beneficial, but a regular habit of moderate exercise for at least 30 minutes on 5 days of the week is recommended for all patients if at all possible, as it is for the general public.

Multifactorial interventions in diabetes

Most existing trial evidence concerns the effect of a single intervention on CVD outcomes. Very few well-designed studies on multifactorial interventions have been published to date. A seminal study in this regard was Steno-2, which provided evidence of the

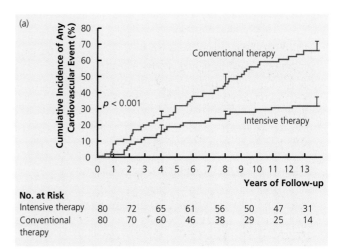

No. at Risk

Intensive therapy	80	72	65	61	56	50	47	31
Conventional therapy	80	70	60	46	38	29	25	14

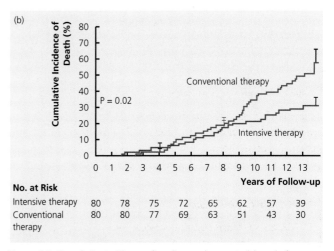

No. at Risk

Intensive therapy	80	78	75	72	65	62	57	39
Conventional therapy	80	80	77	69	63	51	43	30

Figure 5.6 Cumulative incidence of cardiovascular events (a), and of death (b) in the Steno-2 study. Reproduced with permission from Gaede P. *N Engl J Med* 2003;**348**:383–93.

cardiovascular benefits of multifactorial intervention in diabetes (Figure 5.6). One-hundred and sixty type 2 patients with microalbuminuria were randomised to receive conventional treatment in accordance to national Danish guidelines or to an intensive treatment arm. This involved stepwise implementation of behaviour modification and pharmacological treatment that targeted hyperglycaemia, hypertension, dyslipidaemia, microalbuminuria and secondary prevention of cardiovascular disease with aspirin. At the end of the 7.8 year study period there were significant reductions in HbA1c%, systolic and diastolic blood pressure, serum cholesterol and triglycerides, and urine albumin excretion in the treatment group. Patients receiving intensive treatment had a significantly lower risk of cardiovascular disease by about 50%. At the end of the treatment period all the patients were offered intensive treatment and were further followed up for an additional 5.5 years. Despite convergence of most of the risk factors between the groups there was an additional 20% benefit in CVD-related deaths in the original intensive treatment group. This suggests that treatment of multiple risk factors should be started early.

The Alphabet Strategy is an 'ABC of reducing diabetes complications' published in 2002 and is summarised in Boxes 5.4 and 5.5.

Box 5.4 **The Alphabet Strategy**

An ideal management programme should as a minimum address the following issues in the Alphabet Strategy format:

- Advice: Education, self-management, compliance. Special focus on exercise, diet, weight reduction, cessation of smoking
- Blood pressure: Optimal control usually less than 130/80 mmHg, in most cases initial treatment will be with an ACE inhibitor/ARB often in combination with a diuretic
- Cholesterol treatment: Total cholesterol <4.0 mmol/l, LDL <2.0 mmol/l, HDL >1.0 mmol/l and triglycerides <1.7 mmol/l. Statin if cardiovascular disease risk ≥20% over 10 years
- Diabetes control: Ideal HbA1c target 6.5% (48 mmol/mol), metformin first line in most patients. Early recourse to multiple therapy and insulin if targets not reached
- Eye care: Detailed yearly examination and appropriate referral. Aggressive management of vascular risk factors if retinopathy is present
- Feet care: Detailed yearly examination and appropriate referral. Aggressive management of vascular risk factors if neuropathy and peripheral vascular disease is present
- Guardian drugs: Microalbuminuria/proteinuria patients should be considered for ACE inhibitors or ARB. Statins for secondary prevention and primary prevention in those with cardiovascular disease risk ≥20% over 10 years.
- Heart disease/CVD score: To educate patients, guide treatment and as a surrogate clinical audit parameter to analyse the effect of multifactorial intervention

Box 5.5 **Alphabet strategy advice for patients**

1. Do not smoke
2. Maintain ideal body weight for adults (body mass index 20–25 kg/m^2) and avoid central obesity (waist circumference in white Caucasians <102 cm in men and <88 cm in women, and in Asians <90 cm in men and <80 cm in women
3. Keep total dietary intake of fat to ≤30% of total energy intake
4. Keep intake of saturated fats to ≤10% of total fat intake
5. Keep intake of dietary cholesterol to <300 mg/day
6. Replace saturated fats by an increased intake of monounsaturated fats
7. Increase intake of fresh fruit and vegetables to at least five portions per day
8. Regular intake of fish and other sources of omega-3 fatty acids (at least two servings of fish per week)
9. Limit alcohol intake to <21 units/week for men or <14 units/week for women
10. Limit intake of salt to <100 mmol/l day (<6 g of sodium chloride or <2.4 g of sodium per day)
11. Regular aerobic physical activity of at least 30 minutes per day, most days of the week, should be taken (for example, fast walking/swimming)

Table 5.3 Cardiovascular disease outcomes in the CARDS study.

	Placebo (n = 1410)	Atorvastatin (n = 1428)
Type of first event		
Fatal myocardial infarction	20	8
Other acute coronary heart disease death	4	10
Non-fatal myocardial infarction*	41	25
Unstable angina	9	7
Resuscitated cardiac arrest	0	0
Coronary revascularisation	18	12
Fatal stroke	5	1
Non-fatal stroke	30	20
Total	127	83

*Five silent myocardial infarctions included in each group.

Summary

The majority of diabetes care revolves around the prevention of vascular disease. Cardiovascular risk factors must be controlled through a structured programme of regular review if the maximum benefit is to be achieved. Modifiable risk factors include blood pressure, blood glucose, lipids, low physical activity, smoking, proteinuria and renal impairment. Management of risk involves a combination of life-style and pharmacological approaches, tailored to individual patient preferences. Multifactorial intervention packages are the mainstay of preventive care and will typically include a range of drug therapies as well as smoking cessation, nutritional management and regular physical activity.

Further reading

Colhoun HM, Betteridge DJ, Durrington PN, et al. Primary prevention of cardiovascular disease with atorvastatin in type 2 diabetes in the Collaborative Atorvastatin Diabetes Study (CARDS): multicentre randomised placebo-controlled trial. Lancet 2004;**364**:685–96.

National Institute of Health and Clinical Excellence. Diabetes – type 2 (update) CG66. May 2008.

Patel V, Morrissey J. The Alphabet Strategy: The ABC of reducing diabetes complications. Br J Diabetes Vasc Dis 2002;**2**:58–9.

Stevens RJ, Kothari V, Adler AI, et al. on behalf of the United Kingdom Prospective Diabetes Study (UKPDS) Group. The UKPDS risk engine: a model for the risk of coronary heart disease in Type II diabetes (UKPDS 56). Clin Sci 2001;**101**:671–9.

UK Prospective Diabetes Study (UKPDS) Group. Intensive blood-glucose control with sulphonylureas or insulin compared with conventional treatment and risk of complications in patients with type 2 diabetes (UKPDS 33). Lancet 1998;**352**:837–53.

UK Prospective Diabetes Study (UKPDS) Group. Effect of intensive blood-glucose control with metformin on complications in overweight patients with type 2 diabetes (UKPDS 34). Lancet 1998;**352**:854–65.

Ohkubo Y, Kishikawa H, Araki E, Miyata T, Isami S, Motoyoshi S, et al. Intensive insulin therapy prevents the progression of diabetic microvascular complications in Japanese patients with non-insulin-dependent diabetes mellitus: a randomized prospective 6 year study. Diabetes Res Clin Pract 1995;**28**:103–17.

The Action to Control Cardiovascular Risk in Diabetes (ACCORD) Study Group. Effects of Intensive Glucose Lowering in Type 2 Diabetes. N Eng J Med 2008;**358**(24):2545–59.

CHAPTER 6

Management of Blood Glucose in Type 2 Diabetes

Tim Holt[1] and Sudhesh Kumar[2]

[1]Health Sciences Research Institute, Warwick Medical School, University of Warwick, Coventry, UK
[2]Clinical Sciences Research Institute, Warwick Medical School, University of Warwick; and WISDEM, University Hospital, Coventry, UK

OVERVIEW

- Structured education, life-style change, and drug therapy are key to successful glycaemic control in type 2 diabetes
- The majority can be managed in primary care using an expanding range of therapeutic options
- An increasing proportion of patients require insulin to achieve target HbA1c
- Patients should be reviewed every 2–3 months until their personal glycaemic target is achieved, and 6-monthly thereafter

---

Introduction

Rising prevalence of type 2 diabetes and increasing recognition of undiagnosed patients means that each general practice will be regularly making new diagnoses. Most of these patients will not be acutely unwell and some will be asymptomatic and detected on biochemical tests. Modern management of type 2 diabetes involves early effective control of hyperglycaemia through patient education and drug therapy, including insulin if needed. The majority of this can be carried out in primary care, given sufficient practice-based expertise and where necessary, access to secondary care resources.

Whilst there is evidence of safety and efficacy for individual drugs, there is less evidence available on which particular treatment algorithm is most effective for management of type 2 diabetes. Guidelines are therefore based on expert consensus reports rather than robust evidence. Whilst broad principles are similar, there may be significant differences between different guidelines issued by various professional bodies.

Initial management

If a patient has been diagnosed early, with no symptoms or complications and an HbA1c <7% at diagnosis, and if they prefer a time without drug therapy, then an initial 3 months of behavioural adaptation is appropriate. However, a patient with symptoms or a raised HbA1c at diagnosis has probably had diabetes for some time already and there is then a strong case for starting metformin immediately to improve control. There is increasing recognition of the benefits of early blood glucose control on long-term outcomes, a phenomenon that has been termed 'glycaemic memory'.

Life-style advice

This is important throughout the course of diabetes and not just at the start. It should be reinforced at each review even though further drug therapy may be added. Dietary advice and advice on exercise is part of structured education discussed in Chapter 3.

Monitoring HbA1c

HbA1c should be checked every 3 months with action taken each time until the level is below 7% (53 mmol/mol) (or other patient-specific target), and then every 6 months thereafter.

Drug therapy options

In May 2009 the National Institute of Health and Clinical Excellence (NICE) issued a guideline on the use of newer agents for type 2 diabetes, the role of which in management is becoming clearer. Figure 6.1 gives a treatment pathway to guide management.

Key issues in selecting the best option are:

- Metformin is recommended first line for most type 2 patients
- Sulphonylureas have a more immediate effect at reducing blood glucose levels in symptomatic patients and may also be first choice for insulin-deficient individuals
- Sulphonylureas, glitazones and insulin may all cause weight gain and obesity is often already a problem
- Sulphonylureas may put the patient at risk of hypoglycaemia with implications for driving
- There appears to be increased risk of distal fractures in women using glitazones
- Glitazones may cause fluid retention, exacerbating or precipitating heart failure
- Exenatide may assist with weight reduction
- Sitagliptin is licensed for triple therapy (with metformin and a sulphonylurea) but vildagliptin is currently only licensed for use in combination with one of these other agents
- Failure of the HbA1c to respond to exenatide or a gliptin after an appropriate interval requires withdrawal of the drug

---

ABC of Diabetes, 6th edition. By T. Holt and S. Kumar.
Published 2010 by Blackwell Publishing.

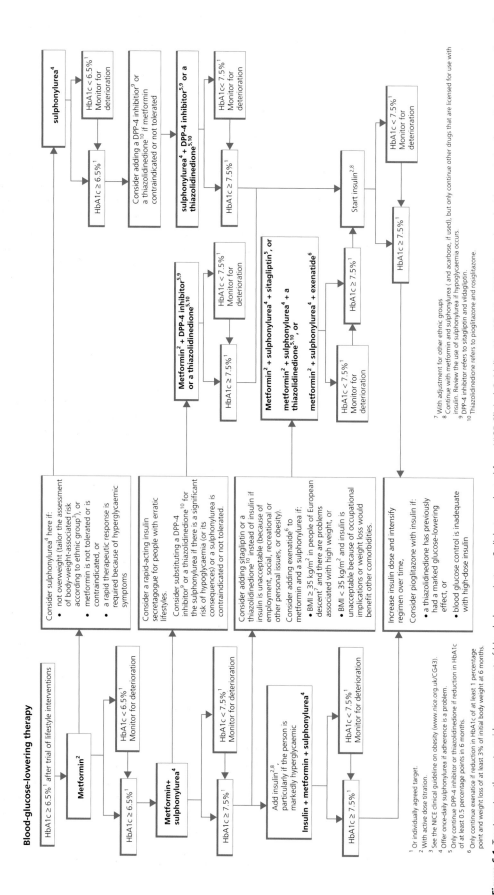

Figure 6.1 Treatment pathway to guide management of blood glucose in type 2 diabetes, adapted from NICE Clinical Guideline No. 87, May 2009. Reproduced with permission from Gaede P. *N Engl J Med* 2008;**358**:580–91.

First line

The majority of patients and certainly those who are overweight (BMI $\geq 25\,kg/m^{-2}$) should start metformin first line. This should be started at 500 mg once or twice a day and the dose increased after 5–7 days (see Box 6.1). Increasing the dose gradually may offset the gastrointestinal side effects that many patients fail to tolerate (Box 6.2).

Box 6.1 **Metformin**

Metformin is now the only available biguanide. Earlier drugs in this group included phenformin, which was withdrawn in the 1970s as it caused lactic acidosis. The biguanides are related to galegine that was originally derived from the French lilac. This plant had been used for centuries to treat the symptoms of diabetes. Metformin is less lipophilic and safer than phenformin, rarely causing lactic acidosis, but is contraindicated in renal failure (see Chapter 12) for this reason. Metformin has a number of beneficial actions in diabetes. It reduces hepatic gluconeogenesis, increases insulin sensitivity and reduces carbohydrate absorption from the gastrointestinal tract. It also improves circulating free fatty acids and very low density lipoprotein (VLDL) levels. The UKPDS study suggested that metformin improves cardiovascular risk independently of its effect on blood glucose levels. Very occasionally, metformin causes reduction in vitamin B12 absorption, and serum B12 levels should be checked in patients taking metformin who develop peripheral neuropathy.

Box 6.2 **Advice from the American Diabetes Association/European Association for the Study of Diabetes on gradual introduction of metformin to avoid side effects**

Initiating metformin therapy (ADA/EASD advice)

1. Begin with low-dose metformin (500 mg) taken once or twice per day with meals (breakfast and/or dinner)

2. After 5–7 days, if gastrointestinal side effects have not occurred, advance dose to 850 or 1000 mg before breakfast and dinner

3. If GI side effects appear as doses advanced, can decrease to previous lower dose and try to advance dose at a later time

4. The maximum effective dose is usually 850 mg twice per day, with modestly greater effectiveness with doses up to 3 g per day. GI side effects may limit the dose that can be used

5. Based on cost considerations, generic metformin is the first choice of therapy. A longer-acting formulation is available in some countries and can be given once per day

---

Non-obese patients may be insulin-deficient (particularly if they have actually lost weight) and could start a sulphonylurea first rather than metformin, but metformin has other benefits and so could be co-prescribed from the start in this situation. The sulphonylurea is titrated upwards according to fasting blood glucose levels if available, or HbA1c. Such patients may need insulin adding early on and their condition should be monitored closely.

Patients starting oral hypoglycaemic therapy in the UK are eligible for free prescriptions. They should be advised to inform the Driving and Vehicle Licensing Authority, who will provide advice on their future responsibilities. This is a legal requirement for patients starting insulin, or those on any sort of treatment who have complications affecting driving ability. Advice to patients about informing the DVLA should be recorded in the medical notes.

Second line

If the HbA1c is still not in target after 2–3 months, offer a second agent. This could either be a sulphonylurea, a glitazone, or a gliptin (see Table 6.1). Glitazones should be avoided in those with, or at risk of heart failure. The short-acting sulphonylurea gliclazide can be given at a dose of 40–320 mg per day (if the slow release version is used, 30–120 mg). Doses above 160 mg should be given as two divided doses. If the patient is unwell or actually losing weight then insulin should be started without delay. This may also be appropriate if the HbA1c is still very high (e.g. over 9%, 75 mmol/mol).

Third line

'Triple therapy' using metformin, a sulphonylurea and either a glitazone or sitagliptin is licensed, but many patients using this combination are candidates for insulin, and this should always be considered before starting a third oral drug. Patients starting insulin can continue their oral medication, but an intensive insulin therapy regimen may be simpler if the sulphonylurea is withdrawn, as the insulin is providing a similar effect exogenously. Patients starting insulin who continue a glitazone are at higher risk of fluid retention and this may precipitate heart failure in susceptible individuals. However, the combination may be beneficial as insulin sensitivity is increased. Glitazones take 8–12 weeks to be effective, and may be added in to improve control in a patient already taking insulin. Most type 2 patients should continue taking metformin unless they fail to tolerate it or develop renal impairment. The patient who is actually *gaining* weight needs more dietary advice. Insulin and sulphonylureas tend to promote weight gain, and the injectible incretin *exenatide* may be useful in this situation but is not licensed for use with insulin. It stimulates glucose-mediated insulin secretion and so does not on its own cause hypoglycaemia. However, the risk of sulphonylurea-induced hypoglycaemia is substantially increased by concomitant exenatide (or gliptin) therapy. See Chapter 19 for more on its mode of action.

Other drug therapies

Other treatment options include the metiglinides (repaglinide or nateglinide), which are taken before a meal to promote insulin secretion and reduce post-prandial hyperglycaemia. Repaglinide is not recommended for use in patients over 75 years old. The alpha-glucosidase inhibitor *acarbose* acts by delaying carbohydrate absorption and can be taken with other agents but is not well tolerated due to its gastrointestinal effects.

Table 6.1 Major classes of hypo-glycaemic agents and their current role in therapy.

Drug class and mode of action	Examples	Advantages	Disadvantages	Place in management
Biguanides: Reduce hepatic gluconeogenesis Increases insulin sensitivity Reduces carbohydrate absorption from the GI tract	Metformin	Weight neutral No risk of hypoglycaemia Possible cardiovascular benefits beyond hypoglycaemic effects Inexpensive	Gastrointestinal side effects limit its usefulness	First line in the majority of patients particularly those with insulin resistance
Sulphonylureas: Increase endogenous insulin production	Gliclazide Glimepiride Glibenclamide	Generally well tolerated Inexpensive Effective at reducing HbA1c and blood glucose in symptomatic patients	Risk of hypoglycaemia Weight gain	Usually second line in patients uncontrolled on metformin alone, but can be used alone in those unable to tolerate metformin or patients who are insulin-deficient
Glitazones: Increase tissue sensitivity to insulin	Pioglitazone (Rosiglitazone)	Usually well tolerated May be used in combination with other oral therapies and with insulin	Take up to 12 weeks for maximum effect Risk of distal fractures in women May cause fluid retention and so precipitate heart failure in susceptible individuals Small degree of weight gain	Usually second line in patients wishing to avoid the more significant weight gain with sulphonylureas, or third line in those still inadequately controlled on two agents (but insulin should be considered in such cases)
Incretin mimetics: Increase the release of endogenous insulin following carbohydrate ingestion Reduce release of pancreatic glucagon Delay gastric emptying	Exenatide Liraglutide	Actually reduce weight Can be used with either metformin, a sulphonylurea, or both	Injectable Expensive Use with sulphonylurea substantially increases risk of hypoglycaemia Nausea and vomiting is common	Could be used second line in a patient wishing to avoid weight gain but can also be added in to a combination of metformin and sulphonylurea
DPP-4 Inhibitors: Delay the clearance of natural incretins	Sitagliptin Vildagliptin	Weight neutral Sitagliptin can be used as triple therapy with metformin and a sulphonylurea	Relatively expensive Not always effective enough at reducing HbA1c	Can be added in second or third line (only sitagliptin licensed for triple therapy)
Meteglinides: Stimulate the release of pre-formed endogenous insulin	Repaglinide Nateglinide	Specifically aimed at post-prandial hyperglycaemia Rapid action	Multiple doses required - before each meal	Repaglinide may be used as monotherapy Nateglinide only licensed for use with metformin
Alpha-glucosidase inhibitors: Delay the digestion and absorption of ingested carbohydrate	Acarbose	Reduces post-prandial hyperglycaemia Weight neutral	Poorly tolerated due to gastrointestinal side effects including flatulence	Can be used alone or in combination with metformin and/or sulphonylurea
Insulin therapy: Direct effect on tissues (particularly muscle and liver) to increase uptake of glucose from plasma	See Chapter 8	Effective at reducing HbA1c	Weight gain and need for high doses in insulin-resistant patients Require regular injection or a pump Risk of hypoglycaemia	Usually commenced when two oral agents have failed to achieve target, but should be considered wherever there are features of insulin deficiency, if control is very poor, or during intercurrent illness to maintain control

Cost effectiveness and other considerations

Treatment choices may be guided by other issues including cost and patient choice. All type 2 patients who can tolerate it should be offered metformin. This drug is inexpensive and was one of the most prescribed medications in the USA in 2006. Insulin therapy is generally the most effective option in terms of HbA1c reduction, but sulphonylureas are cheaper. Glitazones are also relatively expensive, but unlike the latter will not cause hypoglycaemia. This is also an advantage of exenatide and the gliptins, unless

they are co-prescribed with a sulphonylurea. Table 6.1 describes some of the advantages and disadvantages of the individual agents (Figure 6.2).

Starting insulin in general practice

Insulin can be started in most type 2 patients in general practice. As described in Chapter 8, the usual preferred regimen is a twice daily dose of premixed insulin such as Novomix 30 or Mixtard 30

Figure 6.2 Self-monitoring of blood glucose is recommended in all patients taking insulin and may be justified in others on an individual basis.

given before breakfast and before the evening meal. It is usual to start at 6–8 u twice a day with home blood glucose monitoring. The monitoring technique should be taught prior to commencing (and not at the same time as) the insulin. The insulin can then be prescribed and a new appointment arranged to demonstrate the injection technique. In addition to the insulin device, needles (usually 6 mm but longer if the patient is particularly overweight), and a sharps disposal bin should be issued as repeat prescriptions. Needle clipping devices are also prescribable and reduce the volume of sharps requiring disposal. Patients need to be clear about disposal arrangements for their sharps bins when full. The insulin dose can be titrated upwards according to blood glucose levels, usually in increments of 2–4 units, as described in Chapter 8. An alternative is to start with a long-acting analogue such as glargine or detemir at 8 units in the evening, titrating upwards according to fasting glucose

levels. Conversion to a more flexible regimen can be achieved later on, either through the addition of short- or rapid-acting insulins with meals to create a basal-bolus regimen, or by changing over to a premixed insulin twice or three times a day. By this time the patient has become accustomed to injections and any initial needle phobia will have hopefully been overcome. The initial management of a once daily long-acting analogue can usually be managed by general practice teams. Diabetes Specialist Nurses linked to the local hospital diabetes centre are very useful as a source of advice, guidance and patient education, particularly when insulin regimens become more complicated.

Unlike type 1 diabetes, type 2 is a progressive condition in which insulin requirements are likely to increase over time. This should be borne in mind when selecting appropriate intervals to review adequacy of control.

Hypoglycaemia

As discussed in Chapter 5, hypoglycaemia may be seriously detrimental to quality of life and employment prospects. Type 2 patients starting insulin for the first time may or may not have experienced hypoglycaemia before (usually because of sulphonylureas). The risk of this happening is substantially greater with insulin and in some cases this may influence the decision to start insulin over other options, as discussed above. Patients should be counselled over the risk of hypo and given not only practical advice about how to correct it but also a supply of glucagel and glucagon to be used if needed. Risk of hypoglycaemia is the main reason why those taking insulin (unless such treatment is only temporary, i.e. less than 3 months) are legally obliged to inform the Driver and Vehicle Licensing Agency (DVLA). Advice to inform the DVLA should be recorded in the notes. DVLA regulations are revised from time to time and the latest guidance should be consulted.

Figure 6.3 Proportion of patients attaining treatment goals in UKPDS.

Difficulties in achieving targets

Despite concerns about over-treatment, the reality is that too few patients manage to achieve their target HbA1c. Even in the context of a well-organised clinical trial with intensive follow-up such as UKPDS, Figure 6.3 shows the proportion of patients meeting the target HbA1c of <7% (53 mmol/mol). However, patients should be encouraged that all reductions are beneficial.

Further reading

Bailey CJ, Day C. Glycaemic memory. *Br J Diabetes Vasc Dis* 2008;**8**:242–7.

National Institute for Health and Clinical Governance. *Type 2 diabetes – newer agents: short guideline*. Clinical Guideline No. 87, May 2009.

Nissen SE, Wolski K. Effect of rosiglitazone on the risk of myocardial infarction and death from cardiovascular causes. *New Eng J Med* 2007;**356**:2457.

United Kingdom Prospective Diabetes (UKPDS) Group (49). *JAMA* 1999;**281**: 2005–12.

Witters LA. The blooming of the French lilac. *J Clin Invest* 2001;**108**:1105–7.

CHAPTER 7

Hyperglycaemic Emergencies and Management of Diabetes in Hospital

Tim Holt[1] and Sudhesh Kumar[2]

[1]Health Sciences Research Institute, Warwick Medical School, University of Warwick, Coventry, UK
[2]Clinical Sciences Research Institute, Warwick Medical School, University of Warwick; and WISDEM, University Hospital, Coventry, UK

OVERVIEW

- Hyperglycaemic emergencies include diabetic ketoacidosis (DKA) and hyperosmolar hyperglycaemic syndrome (HHS)

- Both require immediate treatment in hospital with insulin and fluid replacement

- In DKA the associated acidosis leads to loss of total body potassium requiring close monitoring and intravenous potassium replacement during rehydration

- Hyperviscosity may lead to thrombosis particularly in older patients with HHS

- Following recovery patients require review of the treatment regimen and close follow-up to prevent recurrence

- Patients admitted to hospital for elective procedures should be managed according to readily available protocols to optimise outcomes

- Involvement of the diabetes specialist team is important when problems arise in hospitalised patients

Introduction

A patient with severe hyperglycaemia can appear to be relatively well, so that potentially life-threatening diabetic ketoacidosis (DKA) or hyperosmolar hyperglycaemic syndrome (HHS) may go unrecognised. Thus, although a patient with significant hyperglycaemia can often be managed quite successfully out of hospital by experienced clinicians, if in doubt it is best to err on the safe side and send the patient to hospital.

Preventing diabetic ketoacidosis (DKA)

When a patient with diabetes presents with an acute illness, one should always assess the glycaemic control. During intercurrent infection, it is necessary for the patient to take larger doses of insulin than usual. Patients are usually taught this but they often require support, especially if they have not dealt with a similar situation before. Often whilst taking antibiotics, the patients may

ABC of Diabetes, 6th edition. By T. Holt and S. Kumar.
Published 2010 by Blackwell Publishing.

have lost appetite and may feel that as they are eating less they should take less insulin. Unfortunately, some patients even stop insulin altogether during illness and this is very likely to lead to diabetic ketoacidosis. If the patient is unable to eat or drink then clearly intravenous fluids and insulin will be required and the patient needs to go to hospital. However, for those patients who are managing an illness at home, regular frequent blood glucose monitoring and additional insulin should be taken as informed by the blood glucose monitoring results. For those taking twice daily pre-mixed insulin, short-acting insulin is valuable, if taken additionally.

Patients who have had diabetic ketoacidosis may also have been given blood or urine ketone meters or ketosticks. These are useful for indicating the onset of ketoacidosis. Sometimes ketoacidosis may be a presenting feature of type 1 diabetes or rarely late in type 2 diabetes.

Clinical features of ketoacidosis

Dehydration and tachypnoea are frequently seen early in DKA. Some clinicians may be able to smell ketone odour on the patient's breath. In more severe DKA, vomiting and drowsiness also develop.

Diagnosis

Blood glucose is typically very high, but is sometimes only modestly raised, especially when the patient has not been eating regularly. In these cases it is important to recognise that the degree of hyperglycaemia is not an index for the severity of the condition. Urine tests for ketones will be positive and plasma ketones will be elevated. Blood gases will show acidosis and reduced bicarbonate. Diabetic ketoacidosis is associated with severe electrolyte abnormalities, particularly of serum potassium. Electrolytes will need to be monitored frequently during the treatment of DKA as there is a net whole-body deficit of potassium and potassium replacement is essential and guided by frequent electrolyte measurements. Full blood counts will usually reveal leukocytosis; however, this does not necessarily imply infection. Similarly, serum amylase is often elevated but does not necessarily indicate pancreatitis. Further investigations are guided by additional clinical features of the particular patient, a chest x-ray is often carried out to exclude a chest infection. Urine analysis and urine culture may be required to exclude urinary tract infection. Blood culture may also be indicated if septicaemia is suspected. The need for further imaging is determined by the clinical presentation.

Treatment

Patients with diabetic ketoacidosis require high-intensity nursing on a one-to-one basis and this is usually achieved in a High Dependency Unit, or if extremely ill and requiring ventilation in an ITU setting.

Fluid and electrolyte management is key to successful treatment of DKA. This is achieved using intravenous saline and the table shows a suitable regimen. Care should be taken in patients with cardiac disease and post-myocardial infarction. In such patients a central venous line and monitoring of central venous pressure (CVP) will be required. Fluid is changed to 5% dextrose once blood glucose has dropped below 11 mmol/l, this will also enable more insulin to be administered as soluble insulin, through a syringe driver and a suitable regime used at the University Hospital, Coventry is shown in Figure 7.1. In severe cases soluble insulin is given IM as a bolus as well. It is important that nursing staff check the equipment regularly as kinks in the line for the fluids or insulin can complicate therapy.

Potassium replacement is nearly always required in patients with DKA, with the possible exception of patients who have advanced renal disease. A suitable regime is also shown in Figure 7.1. Regular urea and electrolyte measurements should be requested and potassium should be maintained between 4-5 mmol/l.

Diabetic Ketoacidosis
This is an EMERGENCY
START INSULIN IMMEDIATELY

Investigations:

U&E's - watch K+
Arterial blood gas
FBC
CXR
ECG
MSU/Cultures

Establish Diagnosis
Please fill inbelow

Time of admission............   ....
Glucose>11.1.....................   ....
Ketones 2+.......................   ....
pH <7.3...........................   ....
HCO3 <15.........................   ....
Hyperglycaemia and DKA are not synonymous

POTASSIUM

wait for initial
K+
add to fluids
as follows

- Serum K+ >5.0
add NO potassium
- Serum K+ 3.5–5.0
add 20 mmol per litre
Serum K+ <3.5
- add 40 mmol per litre

FLUIDS

Approx. 6–10 litres positive
balance in
24 hours (less in
elderly/CCF) -?CVP

Typical fluid replacement
maybe:

1L 0.9% saline 30 minutes

1L 0.9% saline 1 hr

1L 0.9% saline 2 hr

1L 0.9% saline every 4
hours to continue as
indicated by volume status

Change to 5% Dextrose
when glucose <11 mmol/l
If difficulty avoiding
hypoglycaemia use 10%
Dextrose to maintain insulin
in fusion

INSULIN

50 units actrapid to be added to
50 mls N/ Saline to be given
according to sliding scale below.
NEVER STOP INSULIN IN DKA

Finger Stick Glucose	Rate of Insulin In fusion
0.0–5.0	0.5
5.1–7.0	3
7.1–10.0	4
10.1–15.0	5
>15.1	6

Other Measures Consider – NG tube if vomiting/unconscious; urinary catheter to aid fluid balance assessment: CVP line to guide correction of hydration if elderly/heart failure; give antibiotics if infection suspected as a precipitant; anticoagulation may be particularly appropriate in hyperosmoler non-ketotic coma. Administration of bicarbonate is rarely indicated and must only be considered after taking specialist advice.

Please refer ALL patients with DKA/HSS to the Diabetes Team via the Diabetes Centre/Registrar

Figure 7.1 Protocol for the hospital management of diabetic ketoacidosis used at the University Hospital, Coventry.

The acidosis usually corrects itself with fluid replacement and insulin. It is rarely necessary to give bicarbonate, except when the patient has life-threatening acidosis (pH < 6.9) to buy time. When used, 1.26% bicarbonate should be given in 500 ml.

Insulin infusion should be continued until the patient is ready to eat. At this point the patient should be given subcutaneous insulin and after the meal, IV insulin is discontinued. One should aim to ensure patients have ketone-free urine before discharge.

The underlying condition needs to be sought and treated and sick day rules (page 45) should be reinforced to the patient to avoid the same occurring again.

'Brittle diabetes'

A small number of patients have very unstable diabetes that completely disrupts their lives, with repeated admissions to hospital due to either DKA or hypoglycaemia. It is more common in young girls. Often, there are underlying psychological issues that can be quite challenging to manage.

Mismatch of the dose of insulin relative to the patient's diet or exercise should be dealt with. Patients may benefit from learning the technique of carbohydrate counting. Further education through the DAFNE (Dose Adjustment For Normal Eating) programme is also helpful in some cases (see Chapters 3 and 10). If this does not resolve the problem, some of these patients will benefit from continuous subcutaneous insulin infusion through an insulin pump. This requires specialist assessment and management and such patients should be referred to hospital.

Hyperosmolar hyperglycaemic syndrome

These patients often have an extremely high degree of hyperglycaemia without significant acidosis or ketosis. The term 'hyperosmolar hyperglycaemic syndrome' (HSS) is now used in preference to 'hyperosmolar non-ketotic' (HONK) to recognise that a mild degree of ketosis may be present. The management is similar to that of DKA with intravenous fluid and insulin replacement, but such patients often require prophylactic subcutaneous heparin to prevent thrombotic complications. They are less likely to require potassium replacement during rehydration. If hyperosmolarity is so severe that serum sodium is greater than 150, half normal saline is used until serum sodium is below 150 mmol/l. Whilst the biochemical abnormalities in HHS are less complex than in DKA, the condition carries a higher mortality (~15% compared to <5%).

Management of hospitalised type 2 diabetic patients

The management of a type 2 diabetic patient admitted for elective surgery is usually quite straightforward so long as the patient is well controlled. All that is needed is to omit the oral hypoglycaemic agent on the day of surgery and to monitor plasma glucose. If plasma glucose is greater than 11 mmol/l in the morning, IV soluble insulin via an insulin pump will be required. For patients undergoing relatively minor surgery, so long as the operation is done first thing in the morning and the patient is able to eat and drink within an hour of the procedure, this can be accomplished without the need for hospital admission. In this case, it is important that the patient is able to self-manage their diabetes soon after the procedure. Protocols used at the University Hospital, Coventry are shown in Figure 7.1.

Management of diabetes for major elective surgery and type 1 diabetic patients

Such operations are usually managed by intravenous insulin administered using a pump, together with an infusion of 10% dextrose with potassium added in. Regular monitoring of plasma glucose is required and electrolytes should also be measured at least once a day. If blood glucose rises above 11 mmol/l the infusion should be changed to 0.9% saline.

In patients with type 1 diabetes it is important to remember intravenous insulin should not be stopped as such patients can deteriorate very rapidly. Circulating plasma insulin levels rapidly decay if there is no subcutaneous reserve. Conversion to usual insulin regime should be made only when the patient is able to eat and drink normally. Once the subcutaneous insulin injection has been given and the patient has had a meal the IV insulin can be discontinued. If the patient is hyperglycaemic after conversion to subcutaneous insulin additional soluble insulin can be given, but care should be taken to avoid hypoglycaemia at the same time.

Further reading

American Diabetes Association. Hyperglycemic crises in diabetes. *Diabetes Care* 2004;**27**:S94–102.

Singh RK, Perros P, Frier BM. Hospital management of diabetic ketoacidosis: are clinical guidelines implemented effectively? *Diabetic Med* 2004;**14**: 482–6.

Scott A. Hyperosmolar hyperglycaemic syndrome. *Diabetic Med* 2006(s3);**23**: 22–4.

Insulin Therapy

Tim Holt[1] and Sudhesh Kumar[2]

[1] Health Sciences Research Institute, Warwick Medical School, University of Warwick, Coventry, UK
[2] Clinical Sciences Research Institute, Warwick Medical School, University of Warwick; and WISDEM, University Hospital, Coventry, UK

OVERVIEW

- Patients presenting with type 1 diabetes require insulin without delay to avoid ketoacidosis

- An increasing proportion of type 2 patients will require insulin to achieve modern glycaemic control targets

- The majority of type 2 patients requiring insulin can have this treatment initiated in primary care

- A wide range of insulin types is available, but most patients can be managed using a limited selection of regimens and devices

- Familiarity with these devices and regimens overcomes the inertia that may delay the initiation of insulin in type 2 diabetes

---

Introduction

Insulin replacement therapy is essential for a patient with type 1 diabetes and is needed to achieve good glycaemic control in many patients with type 2 diabetes once other agents are no longer able to achieve this effectively. For patients with previously poor glycaemic control insulin has dramatic effects and can enhance wellbeing in a way that other therapies cannot match. Despite these obvious benefits, many patients who have previously taken tablets resist going onto insulin therapy, principally because it is an injectable preparation. Insulin therapy also requires much more active involvement by the patient to adjust the doses. Insulin is unusual as a drug in that the dose different patients take may range very widely from a few units to several hundred units. This often makes healthcare professionals with limited experience wary of managing patients on insulin. The optimal dose is tailored for every given patient and is one that achieves the best possible control avoiding hypoglycaemia as much as possible. In older, frail patients it might be inappropriate to provide intensive insulin therapy and here a once-daily insulin injection that alleviates the symptoms may be all that is required.

Types of insulin

1 **Animal insulins:** Until the 1980s, insulin was manufactured from purified extracts from pancreas of cows and pigs. Today it is manufactured by recombinant DNA technology that involves the insertion of the synthesised genes for insulin into an *Escherichia coli* bacteria, or yeast cells. Resulting protein is yielded in large quantities and then purified. Some patients still use animal insulin, often those individuals who experienced hypoglycaemia after commencing human insulin. Today the vast majority of people with diabetes in the UK use human insulin.

2 **Short-acting insulins:** Short-acting insulin is also known as soluble insulin and has a duration of action of about 6–8 hours and needs to be injected about 30 minutes before meals. Examples are listed in Table 8.1.

3 **Very rapid-acting insulin analogues:** These are newer human insulin analogues that can be taken with or just after the meal because they are absorbed more or less immediately. They are used to cover mealtime hyperglycaemia in a basal-bolus insulin regime that is discussed later.

4 **Intermediate-acting insulins:** These insulins usually have a basic protein like protoamine or zinc added to them to delay their action. They generally tend to have a duration of action of about 8–10 hours after subcutaneous injection. Variants are also available where a duration of action that is considerably longer can be obtained.

5 **Long-acting insulin zinc suspensions:** These are prepared by adding excess zinc ions to insulin and examples of these include ultratard and humulin zinc. These are usually administered at bedtime.

6 **Long-acting insulin analogues:** These insulin analogues provide up to 24-hour basal insulin when injected subcutaneously. These preparations may be suitable for once-daily administration and carry a low-risk of hypoglycaemia because their action profile does not have a 'peak', unlike short-acting or intermediate-acting insulins.

7 **Pre-mixed insulin mixtures:** Several preparations of insulin are available as pre-prepared mixtures in vials or as pre-mixed pens, eliminating the need for patients to mix insulin in a syringe. This reduces the risk of mistakes made while mixing insulin and is also more convenient. Examples of popular insulin mixtures are shown in Table 8.1. The choice of a mixture is dependent on the patient's life-style and meal patterns. Similarly, the selection of particular insulins for a patient is also made bearing in mind the patient's particular circumstances and also their preferences in terms of choice of device, and frequency of injection.

ABC of Diabetes, 6th edition. By T. Holt and S. Kumar.
Published 2010 by Blackwell Publishing.

Table 8.1 Commonly used types of insulin, with examples.

Type of insulin	Examples	Comments
Soluble insulin	Human Actrapid, Pork Acrapid, Humulin S	Actrapid now only available in vials
Rapid-acting insulin analogues	Aspart (Novorapid), Lispro (Humalog), Glulisine (Apidra)	Onset only takes 15 minutes so can be given immediately after, rather than before, a meal when the exact carbohydrate intake is known, if this suits the patient. Short duration of action reduces risk of nocturnal hypoglycaemia and provides flexibility for dose adjustment. Risk of overlap with subsequent injection later in the day is reduced
Long-acting insulin analogues	Glargine (Lantus), Detemir (Levemir)	Have little or no 'peak' of action and are therefore useful as the basal component of the basal-bolus regimen
Isophane (NPH)	Insulatard, Humulin I, Insuman Basal, Hypurine Porcine Isophane, Hypurin Bovine Isophane	Still used as the basal component but does 'peak' in its action. This effect may be useful, but may contribute to the risk of nocturnal hypoglycaemia. Significantly less expensive than long-acting analogues
Biphasic 'pre-mixed' insulins or insulin analogues	Biphasic insulin aspart (Novomix 30), Biphasic insulin Lispro (Humalog Mix25 and Mix50), Mixtard (10, 20, 30, 40, 50), Humulin M3, Insuman Comb (15, 25, 50)	Useful for patients requiring some flexibility but wishing to avoid the more intensive basal-bolus regimen (which requires at least four injections a day). Can be given twice or three times a day before meals. The proportion of overall insulin in the soluble form is indicated by the number. A commonly used option is the '30' strength

Insulin regimens

Starting insulin in type 1 diabetes

Many type 1 patients can start treatment with a twice-daily biphasic regimen, usually about 8 units twice a day and then the dose is optimised. However, in younger patients in particular, a more flexible method is the basal-bolus regime where a long-acting insulin is given at bedtime and meals are covered by soluble insulin or a very short-acting analogue. An increasing number of people in the UK now use insulin analogues, especially if they experience hypoglycaemia on conventional insulins.

Basal-bolus regime

Here an intermediate- or long-acting acting insulin is used at bedtime and meals are covered using a short-acting insulin or a rapid-acting insulin analogue. A long-acting insulin analogue such as insulin glargine or insulin detemir is often used in the UK now as the basal insulin. The timing of the rapid-acting insulin can vary according to the timing of meals. This is convenient for those at work or at college. Rapid-acting insulin analogues have made this regimen more popular because they avoid the overlap effects that may cause problems with frequently administered soluble insulin.

Twice or three times a day biphasic regimen

Some patients opt to have twice-daily biphasic mixtures taken at breakfast and with an evening meal. This can be increased by adding in a lunchtime dose if using a biphasic with a rapid acting component, but there may in some cases be a risk of overlap between the lunchtime and evening doses. Occasionally such patients may require a short-acting or rapid-acting insulin with lunch instead of the biphasic.

Starting insulin in type 2 diabetes

For some type 2 patients where symptom control is the main aim of therapy, and particularly where assistance is required with insulin injections from others, it may be appropriate to provide once-daily insulin injection with a long-acting insulin analogue. For most patients, however, pre-mixed insulin or insulin analogue is preferred. Many patients with type 2 diabetes also elect to go on a basal bolus regimen, which involves four or more injections a day because of the flexibility it offers. For most patients with type 2 diabetes, however, a twice or three times a day regimen of pre-mixed analogues is useful. Maintaining glycaemic control in a patient with type 2 diabetes represents more of a challenge as their needs will change along with disease progression. The doses are increased usually in increments of 2 or 4 units with each dose until glucose control is satisfactory, taking care to avoid hypoglycaemia. This is important to explain to the patient and also to alter insulin doses and the regime as requirements increase. Patients should also be warned about weight gain, particularly in those with type 2 diabetes and concomitant attention to control of obesity is valuable in mitigating this. There is more discussion on insulin management of type 2 patients in Chapter 6.

Administering insulin

In the past most patients used a syringe to draw up and administer insulin. The following modes of administration are now available:

1 *Insulin administered with a syringe*: The patient uses a syringe to draw the appropriate dose from a vial. These plastic insulin syringes are often still preferred by patients who have been using them for years but are less likely to be chosen by patients who start insulin today.
2 *Insulin 'pens'*: These are quite sophisticated and reliable devices and deliver metered doses of insulin either from a cartridge or as a pre-loaded disposable pen that is discarded once the insulin has been fully dispensed. Mixtard 30 is available as a 'InnoLet' device, which may be convenient for patients with visual or manual dexterity problems.
3 *Insulin pumps*: There are now several types of insulin pumps available and the size has reduced so that they are quite unobtrusive. These pumps deliver insulin subcutaneously over 24 hours

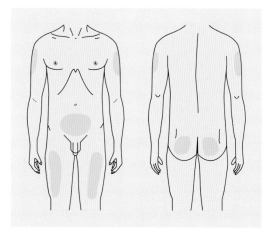

Figure 8.1 Injection sites.

and there are facilities for prandial boosts of insulin. Corrective dose requirements based on carbohydrate intake and the current blood glucose level (entered by the patient) can be calculated by the device and delivered. Insulin pump therapy should be managed by secondary care centres that provide readily accessible expertise to handle any problems. Pump failure may rapidly lead to insulin deficiency with risk of ketosis as the formulation used is rapid acting and has a short plasma half life. Their use is restricted on the NHS to those who cannot be managed otherwise on basal-bolus therapy.

4 *Inhaled insulin:* Inhaled insulin was recently unsuccessfully launched and has been since withdrawn from the market as it did not prove to be as popular as anticipated. Nevertheless newer varieties of inhaled insulins are due on the market. These are of value perhaps only in those patients with severe needle-phobia.

Insulin injection sites

Insulin injection sites that can be used are shown in Figure 8.1. It is most commonly injected in the front of the thigh or on the lower abdominal wall. Patients are advised to rotate sites to reduce the risk of unsightly bruises or fat hypertrophy. Injection sites should be inspected in case lipohypertrophy develops as this can cause instability in glycaemic control, due to variable rates of absorption of insulin.

Insulin injection technique

When the patient first starts insulin he or she is shown how to inject it using the device that has been chosen. The correct dose of insulin is drawn up using the pen and any air bubbles are expelled prior to injection. The length of the needle will also have been chosen for the given patient and the needle should be inserted briskly at 90° to the skin to its whole length. Pressing the plunger rapidly will deliver the dose and the device is then removed.

Problems with insulin injections

Apart from injection site bruises, insulin injections rarely cause problems. Occasionally, insulin allergy may appear and in these cases switching the type of insulin may help. In some cases investigation by skin testing and desensitisation may be needed. Lipohypertrophy at injection sites may occur and it is important to avoid injecting into these areas as absorption is unreliable. Patients who have commenced insulin therapy sometimes experience blurring of vision due to changes in the amount of water in the lens. This usually corrects itself in a few weeks and the patients should be advised not to change their spectacle prescription during this time or to purchase new glasses. Oedema of the feet is also a transient phenomenon and some patients with mild neuropathy may experience a worsening of pain in the feet when starting insulin. This again will improve with time.

Summary

Insulin therapy should where possible be tailored to the needs and preferences of the individual, which differ widely across different patient groups. A need for flexibility is provided for by the rapid-acting insulin analogues that have proven extremely useful for intensive insulin management where life-style patterns and schedules change from day to day. Long-acting insulin analogues have significantly improved the problem of nocturnal hypoglycaemia associated with 'peaking' of the older intermediate-acting insulins. However, for many patients the older insulins are very satisfactory particularly where glycaemic control is not the main issue. For health services there are cost implications with the newer formulations. Optimisation of glycaemic control should, however, be a health service priority given the benefits both in terms of quality of life and avoidance of longer term complications.

Further reading

Bolli GB. Physiological insulin replacement in type 1 diabetes mellitus. *Exp Clin Endocrinol Diabetes* 2001;**109**(Suppl 2):S317–32.

Gallichan M, O'Brien S, Dromgoole P, Nute B, Preston F, Tipson M. *Starting insulin treatment in adults with type 2 diabetes.* Royal College of Nurses, 2004. http://www.rcn.org.uk/__data/assets/pdf_file/0009/78606/002254.pdf

Pickup J, Keen H. Continuous subcutaneous insulin infusion in type 1 diabetes. *BMJ* 2001;**322**:1262–3.

Richter B, Neises G. 'Human' insulin versus animal insulin in people with diabetes mellitus. Cochrane Library, 2005. http://www.mrw.interscience.wiley.com/cochrane/clsysrev/articles/CD003816/frame.html.

Hypoglycaemia

Tim Holt[1], Sudhesh Kumar[2] and Noreen Kumar[3]

[1]Health Sciences Research Institute, Warwick Medical School, University of Warwick, Coventry, UK
[2]Clinical Sciences Research Institute, Warwick Medical School, University of Warwick; and WISDEM, University Hospital, Coventry, UK
[3]St James's Hospital, Leeds, UK

OVERVIEW

- Patients should aim to keep blood glucose levels above 3.9 mmol/l at all times
- Tight glycaemic control increases the risk of hypoglycaemia
- Common causes are too much insulin or sulphonylurea, missed meals or unexpected exercise
- Symptoms may change over time and some may not perceive any symptoms
- Steps should be taken to reduce risk of further episodes of hypoglycaemia by adjusting diet, activity or dose of insulin or sulphonylurea

---

Hypoglycaemic episodes are common and often go unrecognised, potentially leading to severe morbidity. This is most commonly seen in type 1 diabetes, but also occurs in type 2 patients, especially those taking sulphonylureas or insulin. Symptoms can occur at significantly higher blood glucose levels than the usual lower reference range limit of 3.5 mmol/l, particularly in those with long-standing poor glycaemic control. In some patients, the normal protective neurohormonal response to falling blood glucose levels is impaired, thus increasing risk of hypoglycaemia.

Preventing the complications of diabetes is clearly important, and current treatment guidelines recommend near normoglycaemia for most patients. However, tight glycaemic control increases risk of hypoglycaemia as much as threefold, and may be associated with altered cognitive function, seizures or coma. Thus, clinicians must balance the importance of tight control with the potential psychosocial effects that hypoglycaemia may have for the individual. Patients find hypoglycaemia distressing and clinicians should temper their enthusiasm for achieving ideal HbA1c targets by recognising the difficulties this may cause for some people. Treatment goals should be individually negotiated as part of the patient-centred approach.

Causes

Hypoglycaemia most commonly occurs as a result of inadvertent insulin or sulphonylurea overdose, or a change in dose. Other causes

ABC of Diabetes, 6th edition. By T. Holt and S. Kumar.
Published 2010 by Blackwell Publishing.

include a missed or inadequate meal, unexpected exercise or an error in the timing of insulin. Due to the slow absorption and the mealtime peaks of insulin levels, the risk of hypoglycaemia is greatest:

- between meal times
- in the middle of the night, when both soluble and intermediate-acting insulins may be having their peak effect. It may be helpful to reduce the pre-evening meal soluble insulin, and to move the evening intermediate-acting insulin to bedtime. It is essential such patients have a bedtime snack. The use of rapid-acting insulin analogues rather than soluble insulin before meals make nocturnal hypoglycaemia less likely, particularly if teatime is several hours before sleep.

Recently diagnosed type 2 patients may experience episodes of hypoglycaemia several hours after meals. Symptoms in these patients are generally brief.

Some patients are concerned about possible increased hypoglycaemia with human insulin. This is often related to their experience following the switch in the early 1980s from using purified animal (mainly porcine) insulin to human insulin, as the routine treatment of diabetes mellitus. Studies of human insulin have not shown any basis to be concerned that human insulin may cause harm in this way. However, high quality research on patient-oriented outcomes such as quality of life is lacking.

Recognising the hypoglycaemic patient: The clinical picture

Typical symptoms experienced by adults occur as a result of the direct effects of glucose deprivation on the brain, causing neuroglycopenic symptoms such as confusion, drowsiness and difficulty concentrating. Autonomic symptoms result from simultaneous stimulation of the sympatho-adrenal system, leading to sweating, tremor and anxiety.

At every visit, episodes attributed to hypoglycaemia should be discussed. Patients may also experience 'hypos' that go unrecognised. Symptoms are influenced by age. Behavioural changes, including lethargy are common in children, whilst elderly patients are more likely to experience neurological effects such as visual disturbance, loss of balance and incoordination.

Table 9.1. lists some of the common symptoms.

Table 9.1 Common symptoms of hypoglycaemia.

Common symptoms	
CNS	Headache, confusion, difficulty concentrating, personality changes
Cardiovascular	Palpitations
GI	Hunger, nausea, belching
Adrenergic	Sweating, anxiety

Table 9.2 Recognising those at risk of severe hypoglycaemia.

Risk factors for severe hypoglycaemia in diabetes mellitus
Type I diabetes with a history of recurrent severe hypoglycaemia
Young patients
Elderly patients on sulphonylureas
Alcohol
Strenuous exercise in past 24 hours
Critical illness such as sepsis, hepatic, renal or cardiac failure

Although these are the common presenting symptoms, each patient will learn to recognise their own hypoglycaemic episodes, as symptom profiles vary from patient to patient. Some may recognise that certain insulins result in greater hypoglycaemic effects.

Table 9.2. highlights the patients at high risk of severe hypoglycaemia. Patients in these categories need greater vigilance, both in planning the antidiabetic regimen and the acute treatment of hypoglycaemia.

Hypoglycaemia unawareness

A very common problem, which rises in prevalence with increasing duration of diabetes, is the syndrome of 'impaired awareness of hypoglycaemia'. This is the lack of warning symptoms of prevailing hypoglycaemia due to defective epinepherine release and reduced autonomic neural response normally accompanying hypoglycaemia. This condition occurs in about 25% of patients with long-standing disease and is often the result of patients using intensified insulin therapy in order to achieve chronic normoglycaemia. Many of the classical symptoms are either reduced in intensity or lost altogether. This results in a diminished ability to recognise the onset of symptoms, leaving the patient with a significantly increased risk of severe neuroglycopenic hypoglycaemia. This manifests as sudden changes in personality, intellectual function or conscious level without the patient's awareness.

Previous episodes of hypoglycaemia may predispose patients to further episodes. In some patients, it may be that their body no longer recognises low blood sugars as dangerous, and fails to mount a protective response until a more severe level of hypoglycaemia occurs. In these patients a blood glucose level of less than 4.0 mmol/l should be meticulously avoided.

A clue to the patient with reduced hypoglycaemia awareness is a glycaemic profile that includes very low blood glucose measurements. If the patient needs frequently to check their level when it is less than 3.9 mmol/l then it is likely that they have reduced awareness. However, confronting the patient with this assumption in a judgemental way may be destructive to the clinician patient relationship and care is needed, particularly bearing in mind the

implications it may have for fitness to drive. Clinicians have a duty to the rest of society and hypoglycaemia unawareness is a serious development that needs to be 'risk managed' appropriately. If significant and likely to persist, it usually precludes safe driving and the Driver and Vehicle Licensing Authority (DVLA) will need to be informed. In some cases, changes to treatment with improved stability but higher average blood glucose levels may restore hypoglycaemia awareness and the DVLA may then agree to resumption of driving. These decisions need to be openly discussed and well documented in view of the legal implications.

Treatment of the acute episode in adults

Mild episodes can be self-treated by the patient, usually by taking a form of oral carbohydrate containing refined glucose. For example, mild episodes can be treated with glucose tablets or other rapid acting source of glucose.

All forms of refined sugar take approximately 10–15 minutes to relieve symptoms. This delay may result in persisting symptoms that commonly encourage over-treatment, resulting in subsequent hyperglycaemia, triggering a 'vicious cycle'. Symptomatic recovery of hypoglycaemia should be followed by ingestion of complex or unrefined carbohydrate, such as biscuits or breakfast cereal in order to prevent recurrence of the hypoglycaemia. Vigorous exercise and driving should be avoided.

If hypoglycaemia occurs whilst the patient is driving they should pull over and park the car at the earliest safe opportunity, switch the engine off, remove the keys from the ignition, and move out of the driver seat. Driving should not resume until at least 45 minutes have elapsed *after the resumption of a recorded normal blood glucose level*, in view of the potential delay to the return of normal cognitive function.

Treatment of hypoglycaemia is related to duration and severity of the episode. Box 9.1. shows the emergency management of acute hypoglycaemia in adults (British National Formulary).

Box 9.1 **Treatment of hypoglycaemia**

Initial management

- Glucose 10–20 g is given by mouth either in liquid form or as granulated sugar or sugar lumps
- Glucose 10 g is available from 2 teaspoons sugar, three sugar lumps, GlucoGel™ - formerly known as Hypostop™ Gel; milk 200 ml; and non-diet versions of Lucozade™ Sparkling Glucose Drink 50–55 ml, Coca-Cola™ 90 ml, Ribena™ Original 15 ml (to be diluted)

If patient is uncooperative or hypoglycaemia causes unconsciousness

- Glucagon injection 1 mg intramuscularly
- 50 ml of 20% glucose IV infusion
- Infusions of 25 ml of 50% can be given; however, such concentrations are viscous making the infusion more irritant and administration difficult
- Oral glucose should be administered as above once the patient regains consciousness

Glucagon can be used if the patient is at home, or IV access cannot be rapidly obtained. In adults, 1 mg glucagon should be given by intramuscular or subcutaneous injection.

The cause of the hypoglycaemia should always be sought for every episode. The patient's current medication should be reviewed and the appropriate adjustment of insulin dose or hypoglycaemic tablets should be made if necessary. The patient should be advised about common causes of hypoglycaemia such as alcohol and exercise, as well as being educated about the importance of snacks between meals, as well as before and after exercise. For type 1 patients, it may be easy to identify that a hypo has occurred as a result of a miscalculation in the amount of insulin required to balance carbohydrate intake and exercise. Changes in the regular doses may then be unnecessary, and the main lesson learnt may concern the glycaemic effect of the particular carbohydrate source. In type 2 patients taking sulphonylureas, however, the occurrence of hypoglycaemia usually means that a reduction in dosage is appropriate.

Hypoglycaemia in children

Children may not have such dramatic symptoms when having a hypoglycaemic episode, but they may appear unduly lethargic.

Prompt treatment of hypoglycaemia is especially important in children to prevent any subsequent neurological damage. The parent should be advised that a hypoglycaemic episode that causes unconsciousness or fitting is a medical emergency. In the long term, the parents, other carers and the child should be educated about how to recognise the onset of a hypoglycaemic episode. They should always have access to an immediate source of carbohydrate and blood glucose monitoring equipment for immediate confirmation and management of the hypoglycaemia.

The child (depending on the age and ability) should be involved in the management of their condition to ensure greater independence and confidence in the future. When children present with episodes of hypoglycaemia, it is particularly important to ensure the child is taking the correct dose of insulin. If the child finds it hard to adhere to multiple daily injections, twice-daily injection regimens should be offered.

Long-term management of the patient

Greater emphasis on self-management may help patients control parameters that reduce the risk of hypoglycaemia. With the correct education and support, many patients can become expert at managing their disease, ensuring normoglycaemia and minimising the risk of hypoglycaemia. This may be achieved by:

- Basic education in the management of diabetes with constant re-enforcement and support
- A better understanding of concepts such as carbohydrate counting and self-adjustment of the dose of insulin may help reduce risk of hypoglycaemia. The DAFNE programme is discussed on pages 10 and 44
- Objective ways to monitor both the condition and the awareness of hypoglycaemia through blood glucose profiling. As well as traditional self-monitoring, this is now possible through continuous

Figure 9.1 Three-day profile of glucose values sampled every 5 minutes from a patient using an insulin pump, with a different colour for each day, superimposed. This shows a risk of (or actual) hypoglycaemia early in the day, with generally higher values later. Reproduced from Medtronic.

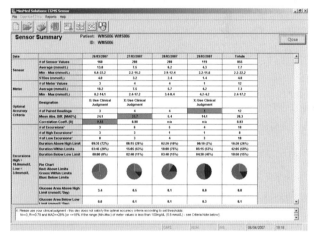

Figure 9.2 The same profile is automatically analysed to identify the proportion of values in range, or in the hypo- or hyperglycaemic ranges (pie chart), as well as mean values by day. Reproduced from Medtronic.

monitoring systems that sample glucose levels subcutaneously every few minutes (see Figures 9.1. and 9.2). However, these are usually only available through outpatient clinics on an occasional basis and not for long-term use at the present time
- Developing the skills to adjust the treatment regime when necessary. This may require protracted training with frequent review, but once achieved may be very empowering and of lasting benefit

Further reading

British National Formulary. British Medical Association and Royal Pharmaceutical Society of Great Britain, London.

British National Formulary for Children. British Medical Association and Royal Pharmaceutical Society of Great Britain, London.

Deary IJ, Frier BM. Glycaemic control in diabetes. *BMJ* 1999;**319**:104–6.

Richter B, Neises G. 'Human' insulin versus animal insulin in people with diabetes mellitus. *Cochrane Database of Systematic Reviews* 2004, Issue 3

Driver and Vehicle Licensing Authority. *At a glance Guide to the current Medical Standards of Fitness to Drive*, available at: http://www.dvla.gov.uk/medical/ataglance.aspx.

Self-Management of Diabetes

Tim Holt[1] and Sudhesh Kumar[2]

[1]Health Sciences Research Institute, Warwick Medical School, University of Warwick, Coventry, UK
[2]Clinical Sciences Research Institute, Warwick Medical School, University of Warwick; and WISDEM, University Hospital, Coventry, UK

OVERVIEW

- The emphasis of modern diabetes care is on self-management, which is appropriate for the majority of patients

- People living with diabetes vary enormously in their individual needs and expectations

- Patients and clinicians should work together to set priorities, define targets, and overcome barriers to quality of life

---

Introduction

The clinic consultation is a valuable but very brief window of opportunity for advice and reflection on progress towards treatment targets. New technologies have increased the availability of clinician advice to patients in ways not foreseen a generation ago. But for the majority of the time patients make their own hour by hour decisions about what to eat, how much insulin to take, and how to adapt this to immediate needs including exercise requirements. Clinicians need to encourage patients to learn self-management skills.

Important issues for the individual include: What should I eat? How should I self-monitor and how frequently? How can I interpret and act on the results of my blood tests to improve control? How can I exercise effectively and safely, to encourage weight loss and improve my health?

What should I eat?

Advice on diet has undergone several significant revisions in the past thirty years. The most recent consensus document was published in *Diabetic Medicine* in 2003 by Connor *et al*. By and large people with diabetes should be encouraged to eat a similar healthy diet as recommended to the general population. However, many patients are unclear about what this actually means in practice (Box 10.1). Patients may believe that they are already eating a healthy diet despite being seriously overweight. The modern approach aims to induce sustainable life-style changes, and avoids the term 'diabetic

diet', but in so doing risks the impression that no therapeutic intervention has been offered at all at diagnosis. This must be avoided through dietary assessment and education, including written materials, and not simply brief verbal 'eat a healthy diet' advice.

Box 10.1 **What does this mean in practice?**

- Use complex carbohydrate as the main energy source rather than fat or protein

- Avoid 'filling up' with fatty foods such as cheese or meat containing high saturated fat levels

- Eat fish, especially oily fish, once or twice a week

- Use olive oil or rapeseed oil in cooking

- Keep sugar to a minimum especially if overweight, although it does not need to be excluded entirely

- Artificial sweeteners are recommended for the overweight and those with hypertriglyceridaemia

- Eat five portions of fruit or vegetables daily

- Restrict salt, which is often present in processed foods

Recommended dietary management for people with diabetes (adapted from Connor, see also Box 10.1)

- Less than 35% of overall energy intake should be made up of fat
- Saturated and trans-unsaturated fat should make up <10% of energy intake
- Daily protein intake should be <1 g/kg of body weight
- 60–70% of total energy intake should consist of carbohydrate and cis-monounsaturated fat
- Up to 10% of overall energy can be in the form of simple carbohydrate (including sucrose) but only in the context of a healthy diet and in the overweight this may prevent weight reduction
- Soluble fibre has beneficial effects on glycaemia and lipids
- Insoluble fibre does not affect glycaemia or lipids but may improve satiety and thereby assist in weight loss
- Encourage foods naturally rich in vitamins and antioxidants - supplements are not usually necessary and in some situations might be harmful
- No more than 6 g sodium chloride daily

ABC of Diabetes, 6th edition. By T. Holt and S. Kumar.
Published 2010 by Blackwell Publishing.

Glycaemic index

Patients may have heard about 'Low GI' diets and wish to try this approach. The glycaemic index (GI) is a measure of how quickly the blood glucose will rise in response to an ingested carbohydrate source. Complex carbohydrate sources have a lower GI than simple sugars. Lists are available of the GI of several hundred foods. There is some evidence that such diets can assist in glycaemic control by smoothing blood glucose fluctuations and improving satiety, assisting in weight loss. However, the measurement of glycaemic index is problematic, and foods may affect glycaemia inconsistently, depending for instance on the other foods consumed. Patients may develop misconceptions about the best food options, and avoid potentially healthy food rich in nutrients such as root vegetables. Low GI diets are therefore not recommended for general adoption, as they do not add much to the standard advice, which also recommends complex carbohydrate as the major energy staple.

Modern nutritional management

The modern focus is on encouraging an interesting, varied diet with regular intake of complex carbohydrate (CHO). Even though such CHO is calorific, it is much less so than an equivalent weight of fat, and tends to satisfy the appetite more effectively as it will be absorbed over a longer period of time. Simple sugars should be kept to a minimum, as they should in the health conscious individual who is aiming to avoid getting diabetes in the first place, but are not completely disallowed and they may in small amounts make the diet more appealing.

The challenge is to reduce calorie intake in a sustainable way, and avoid 'yo-yoing' – as discussed in Chapter 3. For some patients, there is no risk of yo-yoing as the weight simply does not alter following the initial advice. For such patients, a review of the dietary regimen and the written advice provided is necessary. Referral to a dietician may be beneficial (see Box 10.2) and is recommended for all patients at diagnosis.

Box 10.2 **The need for all to understand basic dietary principles**

Dieticians have an important role to play in the team management of diabetes, including the education of patients requiring accurate carbohydrate counting, and for patients with renal failure, coeliac disease, and other conditions often associated with diabetes. However, for many uncomplicated type 2 patients this need not be regarded as a specialist area of dietetics. Doctors, nurses and other professionals must feel able to reinforce the recommended advice. Familiarity with the principles of a healthy diet and the ability to translate this into practical meal suggestions should be within the toolkit of all health professionals. The entire team should have access to the same printable educational material so that a consistent message can be provided repeatedly if needed. Online resources have helped a lot in facilitating this (see Chapter 20)

A few additional points of advice may be helpful to supplement the 'healthy eating' message:

- Fruit is recommended on a regular basis, but *fruit juice* is surprisingly high in carbohydrate and calories as it is often made from concentrate
- Muesli is generally considered a healthy food, but often contains a lot of sugar and raisins that are a very concentrated form of carbohydrate, and unlike some other foods that may be taken occasionally, muesli is eaten every morning by some patients. A bowl of shredded wheat or some wholegrain toast are preferable as regular alternatives
- Patients sometimes take away with the 'healthy eating' message an assumption that drinks such as cola and lemonade are 'healthier' than their low calorie equivalents, as they are less likely to contain artificial ingredients. In fact such drinks are loaded with simple carbohydrate and their exclusion may help very significantly in reducing calorie intake, and blood sugar levels. Some patients may have been self-treating the thirst of hyperglycaemia with these drinks prior to diagnosis. Low calorie alternatives containing no carbohydrate at all are now widely available and generally safe. (The exception is that people with phenylketonuria should avoid aspartame, which contains phenylalanine)
- Food should remain interesting. A simple piece of advice is to encourage patients to ensure their plate contains foods of several different colours (a 'rainbow', see Chapter 20)
- Salad foods are available all the year round, and should not be viewed as exclusively a summer option
- Whilst most foods can be taken at least 'occasionally', there is a danger that patients may consume a different 'occasional treat' item on each day of the week, believing (correctly, in a sense) that they have followed the advice. This may be one reason why a patient fails to lose weight
- Processed foods including sauces often contain a lot of added salt, which manufacturers know will make them more likely to sell. The 6 g/day limit is on sodium *chloride*, and this equates to 2.4 g of sodium, as salt is only 40% sodium. This is important, as manufacturers often give the content simply as sodium, which does not sound as high

Alcohol

Alcohol is not excluded in diabetes, and in moderation carries some cardiovascular benefits, but the following issues are very important:

- Many alcoholic drinks are highly calorific, partly because the alcohol itself is so, even when not combined with sweet ingredients
- Sweet alcoholic drinks include sherries and liqueurs, which not only contain calories but also sugar that is likely to raise blood glucose levels
- The same applies to beers, even 'bitters', particularly the darker ones
- Lagers, or dry wines in strict moderation are therefore preferable
- Intoxication with alcohol may impair an individual's ability to control their diabetes, for instance through their decision making over carbohydrate intake and insulin doses
- Alcohol may mask the symptoms of hypoglycaemia – the patient who is actually hypo may not receive assistance as it is clear they are intoxicated

Figure 10.1 Alcohol should be taken only with awareness of the risks, which are higher in those with diabetes. Reproduced with permission from Getty Images.

- Alcohol directly impairs the metabolic response to falling blood glucose
- Alcohol interacts with sulphonylureas to increase the risk of hypoglycaemia
- A combination of hypoglycaemia and alcohol intoxication puts the patient at risk of a seizure

Individuals who wish to take alcohol need to be aware of all of these issues. A particularly dangerous situation is where insulin is taken at a social event, as well as alcohol, followed by delay in the arrival of the meal, leading to severe hypoglycaemia that is not recognised early enough by the intoxicated patient or his/her companions. It is often at social events where the individual loses control of meal arrangements (content and timing), and at the same events alcohol is frequently on offer (Figure 10.1).

Should I self-monitor?

In the UK, there is a national funding issue over self-monitoring, as testing strips are still quite expensive and are prescribed under the NHS. Most patients with diabetes get free prescriptions, and the cost of this activity is therefore borne largely by the state. In countries without such a system, the cost is likely to fall on the individual, and any benefits may then add to health inequalities between socio-economic groups.

In selecting patients likely to benefit from self-monitoring, the following issues should be considered:

Treatment regimen: Those taking insulin (particularly type 1 patients) are far more likely to benefit than patients treated with life-style measures alone or oral medication, for reasons discussed below. Type 1 patients are generally recommended to monitor at least twice a day. The DiGEM study (Farmer *et al.* 2007) found that self-monitoring in people with non-insulin treated type 2 diabetes not only failed to improve glycaemic control, but also failed to improve psychological parameters such as quality of life

Symptom awareness: Some patients are better than others at predicting their current blood glucose level without monitoring, and may be able to predict whether it is likely to be rising, falling or static. Those who have lost hypoglycaemia awareness are particularly dependent on frequent monitoring. Others may tend to mistake normal symptoms (e.g. of hunger or anxiety) for hypoglycaemia

The need for flexibility: For some patients, flexibility in carbohydrate intake and exercise is required for their life-style, which might include frequent international travel, night-shifts, or unpredictable delays in mealtimes. Such influences should not be encouraged as they are likely to be disruptive, but if they are unavoidable then frequent monitoring combined with appropriate adjustments may maintain stability. Patients driving for long distances and at any risk of hypoglycaemia should generally monitor before setting off and every 90 minutes during the journey. For patients wishing to fast during Ramadan, self-monitoring is often recommended during this period

Response to abnormal results: It is part of the personality of some patients to 'over-react' to abnormal results. Such individuals, unless they can 'retrain' this tendency, are at risk of 'tampering,' i.e. of worsening rather than improving control as a result of the monitoring. It is sometimes possible to identify such a predisposition among the behaviours of the patient in other areas of their life

Other psychological issues: 'Learned helplessness' is a potential psychological effect of self-monitoring in the patient who has not been taught (or is unable to learn) to respond appropriately to self-monitored results. It is in a sense the *opposite* of self-efficacy. Unexpected fluctuations become perplexing and demoralising. This may reduce quality of life and can easily result if self-monitoring is recommended with no training in responding behaviourally to the results

Continuous glucose monitoring devices

Figures 10.2 and 10.3 represents a profile from a type 2 and a type 1 patient respectively, using a continuous glucose monitoring device taking subcutaneous glucose measurements every 5 minutes for 72 hours. A subcutaneous probe is inserted under the skin. Such devices are now available to allow patients and clinicians to explore underlying patterns in blood glucose profiles, but the technology is still quite expensive for routine use.

How should I use my blood glucose results to improve control?

Chapter 3 discussed the now established principle of patient autonomy, in succession to the more paternalistic approach of the past. This paternalism arose at a time when self-monitoring at home was not a practical proposition - the technology had simply not been invented. Patients depended much more on a doctor's advice to achieve glycaemic control, and might need admission to hospital to

Figure 10.2 Profile from a patient with type 2 diabetes treated with metformin only. Fluctuations are relatively small and the fasting level is very similar on each of the days sampled. Reproduced from Medtronic.

Figure 10.3 Profile from a patient with type 1 diabetes treated with an insulin pump. The HbA1c is similar to that in Figure 10.2. but the dynamical properties are clearly different. Reproduced from Medtronic.

measure the diurnal profile over a period of days. This approach is still required in difficult cases, including the more brittle patterns seen in children.

Self-monitoring technology has changed this situation, as a patient can now easily build such a profile through regular monitoring in the more natural environment of their usual daily activities (see Box 10.3).

Box 10.3 **Retrospective and prospective approaches**

The interpretation and analysis of self-monitored results should be tailored to the patient's needs and the type of diabetes and treatment regimen. There are a number of possible strategies. Patients may:

- Build a profile, in tabulated or graphical form, to examine retrospectively either alone, or in consultation with a practitioner
- Take readings purely to influence immediate actions prospectively, e.g. to detect and avoid imminent hypoglycaemia or as a precaution before driving

---

- A combination of the two
- Take an occasional sporadic reading to check that the system has not moved 'too far out'
- Reserve self-monitoring for episodes of acute illness

This list suggests a distinction between retrospective and prospective approaches. Each has its benefits and limitations

Retrospective analysis

The traditional approach aims to identify patterns that are only evident when several days or more of data are gathered continuously. This may improve understanding of the dynamical behaviour. Software is available to enable sharing of the data between patient and clinician via the internet (see Figure 10.5). However, there are several limitations of this approach.

First of all, the profile may be 'complete,' but significant excursions may occur between monitoring (see Figure 10.4). Carbohydrate intake and insulin doses may be recorded much less consistently than the glucose data, and exercise is very difficult to quantify. Data may be uploaded to a personal computer to assist with processing and statistical evaluation, but more often the raw data are presented without any such tools. The human eye struggles to perceive patterns in numerical data, particularly when decimal places are used, which is why graphical displays may be very helpful.

Secondly, the assumption is often made that the profile has been gathered without the emerging results influencing the patient's behaviour, as it might if we were collecting it during a study on an animal, or during a 'blinded' monitoring exercise. But the patient's responses to the readings may be a powerful determinant of the dynamical behaviour. High fasting levels may arise through over-correction of nocturnal hypoglycaemia, for instance, but such details may not be recorded in the profile.

Despite these limitations, the following guidelines may help improve control based on retrospective analysis of the profile.

Figure 10.4 Increase in blood glucose after breakfast on each of the three monitoring days during a continuous glucose monitoring system (CGMS) recording. A self-monitoring schedule involving measurements four times a day (before each meal and at bedtime) would have missed these excursions. Reproduced from Medtronic.

Advice based on the retrospective approach (adapted from 5th edition of the ABC of Diabetes)

Unless there is good reason to alter doses acutely (such as imminent hypoglycaemia or intercurrent illness), for most patients it is best to keep doses fairly stable (with less than 10% change) from day to day. Patterns of variation are more important than single random glucose values.

Examine the profile and attempt to identify consistent, *reproducible* peaks and troughs.

To increase blood glucose in the troughs:

- Eat more carbohydrate at or before the times when blood glucose values are at their lowest, usually at mid-morning and at bed-time
- Reduce the dose of insulin before the trough
- Consider changing a short acting insulin to a rapid acting insulin analogue to avoid pre-meal hypoglycaemia

To decrease blood glucose in the peaks:

- Reduce carbohydrate intake at the meals that precede the peaks
- Increase the dose of insulin before the peak

These adjustments should be made with an awareness of the duration of action of the various types of insulin (see Chapter 8).

To decrease fasting hyperglycaemia:

- Increase the evening intermediate or long acting insulin
- If this causes nocturnal hypoglycaemia, consider splitting the pre-dinner insulin into two parts, with the short or rapid acting insulin before dinner and the longer acting insulin at bedtime. Alternatively, if the patient is taking an intermediate acting insulin in the evening, consider changing to a long acting insulin analogue such as detemir or glargine.

To reduce nocturnal hypoglycaemia:

- Reduce the dose of the evening intermediate insulin or long acting insulin analogue
- Advise the patient to take carbohydrate at bedtime. This is particularly important if the bedtime blood glucose level is <6.0 mmol/L
- Consider changing evening intermediate acting insulin to a long acting insulin analogue, to avoid nocturnal 'peaking' of insulin levels.

Software programmes have been designed to assist in dose adjustment to optimise insulin regimens. These include the CoPilot system (see Figure 10.5).

The prospective approach

In the past the retrospective approach was promoted as the only appropriate technique, but may seem like 'driving a car by looking through the rear mirror', to quote one patient. This is a particular problem if life-styles require flexibility and immediate needs are inconsistent from one day to the next. To continue the metaphor, patients are likely to want to use the front windscreen *prospectively* as well as the rear mirror retrospectively, but there are dangers if the patient is not sufficiently skilled at this.

Figure 10.5 The 'CoPilot' programme for assisting in management of diabetes. Reproduced with kind permission from Abbott Laboratories Limited.

Some of the problems with prospective responses to blood glucose results include:

- **'Chasing the tail':** Displacement of the glucose level is detected, but the response is to over-correct, resulting in displacement in the opposite direction. This may again lead to over-correction, repeating the cycle, and so on
- **Overlap of insulin doses:** Self-monitoring may occur before the most recent insulin dose has taken full effect, so that a high blood glucose level is treated with an unnecessary corrective dose, when restoration of a normal level would have occurred without any interference
- **Inappropriate adjustment of long-acting insulin:** In another common scenario, the patient detects a raised measurement prior to the daily long-acting insulin dose, and increases the long-acting dose accordingly. This action is delayed, and then overlaps with other insulin doses hours later or the following day
- **Inappropriate response to a non-significant fluctuation in the glucose level:** As Figure 10.3 demonstrates, glucose levels may fluctuate quite widely over a period of an hour or two, and some of this fluctuation represents dynamical 'noise' that should be ignored rather than used as a basis for prospective action. Impulsive responses to such noise will worsen control

These problems are typical of the 'tampering' phenomenon, in which self-monitoring results in deterioration rather than improvement in control, justifying past caution over this prospective

Figure 10.6 The retrospective and prospective approaches should ideally complement each other. After all, no good driver attempts to control the vehicle without using both the windscreen and the rear mirrors.

approach. But the modern patient is likely to want to develop prospective control skills to provide flexibility (Figure 10.6). The DAFNE approach (Box 10.4) involves an individually tailored algorithm for dose adjustment, combined with accurate carbohydrate counting. There is no dietary restriction, and insulin doses are adapted to carbohydrate intake choices. It is the only evidenced-based programme currently on offer for type 1 patients wishing to adjust doses flexibly. An adapted programme for the 11–16 year age group is under development.

Box 10.4 **DAFNE**

DAFNE ('Dose Adjustment For Normal Eating') is a 5-day training programme for adults with type 1 diabetes. It involves accurate carbohydrate counting and adjustment of insulin doses according to need. It is suitable for well-motivated patients who have been diagnosed for at least 6 months, and who are prepared to monitor four to six times a day and inject insulin frequently. It is based on the idea that tailoring insulin doses to the person's usual diet (which is in principle unrestricted) is the best way of achieving glycaemic control without increased hypoglycaemia. It has been shown in a randomised controlled trial to improve HbA1c levels (as well as quality of life scores) without increasing the frequency of severe hypoglycaemia. It is not known whether in the long term metabolic outcomes are affected by the dietary freedom, but short-term cardiovascular risk factors were unaffected. The details of the DAFNE approach are not widely available as it is important that patients using this technique are properly trained by attending the 5-day course. For the reference to the DAFNE trial report, see Chapter 3. For details on how to apply or refer, see: www.dafne.uk.com

---

Self-monitoring techniques

There is now a wide variety of self-monitoring systems available. It is preferable for the whole health care team to be familiar with the same device or a small number of alternatives.

Whilst the devices are not themselves prescribable in the UK, manufacturers will usually supply them free of charge to diabetes teams (e.g. general practices or hospital diabetes centres) to distribute to patients. The testing strips can then be prescribed. The monitors must be user-friendly in a range of environments and the best options will provide the following features:

- Small, compact, and easily carried in clothing or a handbag
- Only require a small amount of blood for a measurement
- Beep to confirm that sufficient blood has been applied, but not so loudly that monitoring cannot be done discreetly
- Give an accurate reading in a short time frame e.g. 12 seconds
- Do not require blood to be 'wiped off' the end of the strip
- Have a luminescent screen and so usable in the dark
- Use testing strips that can be disposed of by flushing away
- Preferably include the option of testing for blood ketones
- Have a memory for recall of past results
- Increasingly, patients will want to upload results to a personal computer for retrospective analysis, a feature available with some but not all devices

Blood may be taken from the distal edges of the fingers (the central pulp of the fingers should be avoided to preserve nerve ending function in the long run), from the forearms (less pain sensitive) from the thenar or hypothenar eminences (see Figure 10.7), or from the ear lobes (which are usually very vascular and bleed easily even when other sites do not).

Ideal frequency of self-monitoring

The expected benefits and frequency of self-monitoring should be agreed between patient and clinician before starting. Patients on insulin whose diabetes is intensively (and 'prospectively') managed will need to monitor four to six times per day to gain maximum benefit, particularly when flexibility is required. Other patients, including those with type 2 diabetes whose carbohydrate intake is relatively constant in quantity and timing will require readings less often, provided hypoglycaemia awareness is intact. For patients who are not taking insulin but in whom it has been decided that monitoring is beneficial, a measurement taken twice a week may be appropriate, increased during illness. Those taking oral medication (and certainly those taking insulin) may benefit from monitoring before driving – a policy recommended by the Driving and Vehicle

Classical finger-prick areas. The tips and pulp of the fingers should be avoided to preserve sensitivity. Choice of site should be rotated.

Alternative areas for blood sampling. These areas are less painful and may improve acceptability particularly in children, but the blood glucose mesasurements respond more slowly following carbohydrate ingestion, particularly at the forearm.

Figure 10.7 Sites on the hand suitable for blood sampling.

Licensing Authority. Insulin users should monitor before setting off and every 90 minutes during the journey. Ramadan is a situation when individuals who do not usually monitor may benefit from doing so. Frequency of self-monitoring should be increased at times of sickness, particularly for type 1 patients (Box 10.5).

Box 10.5 **Sick day rules**

Glycaemic control may become very difficult during intercurrent illness, particularly when vomiting occurs. The basic principles are to monitor frequently (every 2–4 hours), not to stop insulin (as more than the usual dose is typically needed), to titrate insulin doses to blood glucose results, and to maintain a regular intake of easily digested simple carbohydrate. If this is not possible, admission to hospital is needed. Regular testing of the urine or blood for ketones during the illness is useful to detect the onset of ketoacidosis, which requires prompt treatment with intravenous fluids and insulin.

New technologies

The past 15 years have seen a rapid development of technologies to assist patients in self-management. These include computer assisted self-management programmes and flow sheets, telemedicine options, Internet-based educational software, and automated telephone products. In a systematic review in 2006 Jackson and colleagues found that as well as improvements in HbA1c reported in most studies, IT-based interventions improved health care utilisation, behaviours, attitudes, knowledge and skills. However, ethnic minorities are not well represented in the research literature, and unless the problem of access is addressed the development of such technologies is likely to widen rather than reduce health inequalities.

Maintaining an active life-style

Physical activity and diabetes

Regular moderate aerobic physical activity for at least 30 minutes on 5 days of the week, recommended for the whole population, is particularly valuable in those with diabetes. Generally speaking, the activity should be sufficient to make the person breathless and raise the heart rate. This activity should:

- increase the chances of sustained weight loss
- improve the lipid profile
- reduce blood pressure

It also increases insulin sensitivity and can improve glycaemic control, provided appropriate account is taken for the exercise in adjusting insulin doses and carbohydrate intake. Increasing the exercise beyond a moderate level is likely to result in little further benefit and may be risky. The risks are not only those of hypoglycaemia (particularly in insulin-treated patients) but also of actual physical injury. A sprained ankle is easily gained and may preclude exercise for several weeks. Cardiovascular benefits are not sustained for long after an exercise programme ceases, and regular moderate activity is far more beneficial than unprepared excessive exertion. Like crash dieting, such behaviour is counter-productive and should be discouraged.

For some patients, obesity and associated arthritis or other physical problems may make exercise difficult or impossible. Advice and guidance is now widely available through personal trainers, but such people must be adequately trained themselves. Swimming is a usually safe and effective form of exercise, as is brisk walking. For those who cannot manage this, any amount of physical activity, however small, is better than nothing and some people may be able to increase their activity significantly simply by rearranging their work environment. Using a toilet on a different floor, avoiding using the lift, walking to visit others in different office rooms rather than telephoning, and other simple changes to everyday habits may be very beneficial.

Summary

The emphasis of diabetes care is on self-management, but the availability of medical expertise is as important as ever. Patients need to be taught a range of skills in order to take control and 'ownership' of their condition. These include advice on nutritional management and exercise to achieve sustained weight loss and improved cardiovascular risk, and training in managing blood glucose levels through self-monitoring where appropriate. Through these measures the patient can work together with the health care team to develop the confidence and self-efficacy to overcome the day to day challenges of diabetes.

Further reading

Farmer A, Wade A, Goyder E, et al. Impact of self monitoring of blood glucose in the management of patients with non-insulin treated diabetes: open parallel group randomised trial. *BMJ* 2007;**335**:132 (21 July), doi:10.1136/bmj.39247.447431.BE

Jackson CL, Bolen S, Brancati FL, et al. A Systematic Review of Interactive Computer-assisted Technology in Diabetes Care. *J Gen Int Med* 2006;**21**:105–10.

Connor H, et al. Nutritional Subcommittee of the Diabetes Care Advisory Committee of Diabetes UK. *Diabetic Medicine* 2003;**20**:786–807.

Department of Health. *The expert patient: a new approach to chronic disease management for the twenty-first century.* London: Department of Health, 2001; www.ohn.gov.uk/ohn/people/expert.

Tattersall R. The expert patient: A new approach to chronic disease management for the twenty-first century. *Clin Med JRCPL* 2002;**2**:227–9.

CHAPTER 11

Surveillance for Complications

Tim Holt[1] and Sudhesh Kumar[2]

[1]Health Sciences Research Institute, Warwick Medical School, University of Warwick, Coventry, UK
[2]Clinical Sciences Research Institute, Warwick Medical School, University of Warwick; and WISDEM, University Hospital, Coventry, UK

OVERVIEW

- Early detection of complications requires a systematic surveillance programme involving regular review, examination and blood monitoring
- Complications particularly amenable to early detection include retinopathy, microalbuminuria and foot ulceration risk
- Surveillance also provides opportunities for review of control of the key cardiovascular risk factors: glycaemia, blood pressure and lipids
- Regular contact facilitates discussion on factors affecting quality of life including mood, hypoglycaemia, erectile dysfunction and driving safety

---

Introduction

Once the diagnosis of diabetes is confirmed, the patient should be entered into a structured programme of surveillance and follow-up. The purpose of surveillance is twofold: to identify the development of complications as early as possible and to address factors the treatment of which will prevent or delay their onset. The importance of this programme must be clearly explained as part of the initial patient education, emphasising its benefits and strong evidence base.

Structure of a basic surveillance programme

This chapter describes the techniques used to conduct diabetes surveillance (Box 11.1). Treatments and targets are discussed elsewhere in the book. Most of the surveillance measures required should be conducted at least annually. As discussed in Chapter 18, a regular habit of annual review is important both to improve concordance and to ensure that the process is completed. If some of the measures are taken opportunistically outside the annual review appointments then this may reduce the effectiveness of the programme, as the patient may be less inclined to attend for the remaining checks. However, blood pressure, glycaemic control and

monitoring of renal function often need to be carried out more frequently, outside the annual reviews.

Box 11.1 **Minimum surveillance measures for diabetes**

- Weight and body mass index
- Blood pressure measurement
- Serum cholesterol estimation
- Glycosylated haemoglobin (HbA1c)
- Estimated glomerular filtration rate (e-GFR)
- Foot examination
- Digital retinal photography
- Urinalysis for microalbumin
- Depression screening

Weight and body mass index

Weight is a good index of the success of life-style change. Ninety percent of patients with type 2 diabetes are overweight or obese at diagnosis and benefit from weight reduction, particularly when this is associated with increased physical activity. Abdominal obesity carries a particularly raised risk of cardiovascular disease, so waist measurement is also useful to monitor success in reducing this risk factor. The patient should usually be weighed with coat and shoes off but otherwise clothed, on regularly calibrated scales, and preferably the same scales each time (Figure 11.1).

Blood pressure measurement

Blood pressure should be taken with the patient sitting down and after a few minutes rest, with the cuff at the same level as the heart and the elbow very slightly flexed. An appropriate sized cuff is important, as too small a cuff will give falsely raised readings. Initially it is worth checking the blood pressure in both arms, and if there is consistent difference then the arm with the highest pressure should be used in future for monitoring. It is also useful to measure the sitting and standing blood pressure, and this should be done annually particularly in elderly patients. A fall of greater than 20 mmHg after standing may be a sign of autonomic neuropathy (see page 73). If such a fall is associated

ABC of Diabetes, 6th edition. By T. Holt and S. Kumar.
Published 2010 by Blackwell Publishing.

Figure 11.1 Weight measurement at the University Hospital, Coventry. The black mat on the floor in the background is a device for measuring very heavy patients over 200 kg.

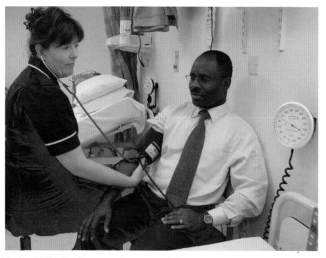

Figure 11.2 Blood pressure measurement.

with postural hypotension symptoms this will affect blood pressure management and may be a contraindication to drug therapy. Alternatively, it may be associated with one of the drugs currently used to reduce blood pressure in which case it may resolve when this drug is stopped or changed to an alternative. Beta blockers, thiazide diuretics and alpha blockers are particularly likely to cause postural hypotension.

Cholesterol and lipids

Patients should ideally have a fasting lipid profile measured annually, to include total serum cholesterol, HDL, LDL and fasting triglycerides. The majority of patients should be prescribed a lipid-lowering agent (see Chapter 5) irrespective of their baseline serum cholesterol. It will therefore usually be advisable to check the liver function tests on at least an annual basis.

Glycosylated haemoglobin (HbA1c)

The HbA1c is a reflection of average blood glucose values over the previous 2–3 months. In the past the value has been given as a percentage, which is *not* equivalent to a glucose value (frequently causing confusion). This is the percentage of haemoglobin A that has become glycosylated by exposure to plasma glucose during the lifespan of the red blood cells. The new IFCC units for HbA1c reporting discussed in Chapter 1 should resolve this confusion. Measurement should be made every 6 months, or at the very least annually. There is little point in repeating the measurement earlier than 2 months following a change in therapy, as it takes this long to change in response to red blood cell turnover. Other means of gauging control (including self-monitored blood glucose levels and symptoms of hypoglycaemia), may be used in the meantime to guide decisions on treatment.

Estimated glomerular filtration rate (e-GFR)

Whilst at best an approximation, this marker is a much more adequate index of renal function than serum creatinine, as it takes account of age, sex and ethnicity. In the UK, the e-GFR can be requested on a blood sample at the same time as the urea, electrolytes and creatinine, and is calculated automatically by the laboratory using the MDRD formula (although the adjustment for ethnicity is not included). The e-GFR should be measured at least annually, and more frequently in patients whose renal function is reduced or at risk of declining, in those taking medication that can affect renal function such as diuretics, non-steroidal anti-inflammatory drugs, or ACE inhibitors, and those taking drugs that are contraindicated if renal function is poor (such as metformin). Abnormal renal function may influence the choice of statin (see page 55). Such decisions are much more securely based on e-GFR than on serum creatinine measurements.

More than one e-GFR measurement is required to confirm renal impairment, and unexpectedly low values should be followed up by repeated measurements to confirm (as well as to exclude progressive decline), as levels may be artificially reduced in the short term by dehydration, recent changes in medication, or other factors. To maximise the validity of an e-GFR measurement, the patient should avoid ingesting meat for 12 hours before the blood sampling.

Foot examination

All patients with diabetes should have a thorough foot examination at least annually, and in those with signs of complications or 'at-risk' features this frequency should be increased. The examination should include, as a minimum, the following:

- **Inspection of the general health of the feet:** signs of deformity, hair loss, loss of skin integrity, loss of sweating, swelling of joints, callosities, nail health, fungal infection between the toes. Deformity or swelling may suggest an underlying Charcot's neuroarthropathy (see Chapter 14). Callosities suggest abnormal distribution of weight over the sole, which may indicate peripheral neuropathy.

Figure 11.3 Identifying pedal pulses using a Doppler device at the University Hospital, Coventry. Photograph courtesy of Mr G Deogan.

Figure 11.4 At risk areas for peripheral neuropathy and neuropathic ulceration.

- **Assessment of vascular sufficiency:** temperature of the skin, detection of dorsalis pedis and posterior tibial pulses, capillary return at the toes. A Doppler device (Figure 11.3) may assist in assessing vascular sufficiency, particularly when used in experienced hands to measure ankle brachial pressure index, but if the pedal pulses cannot be detected manually then the arterial supply should be considered abnormal.
- **Assessment of neurological integrity:** light touch sensation using a 10 g nylon microfibre device at all of the 'at-risk' areas (see Figure 14.6) and vibration sense at the great toe and ankle; Achilles tendon reflex (Figure 11.4).

Advice and treatment of foot complications is covered on pages 64-71.

Digital retinal photography

Traditional fundoscopic examination, even in experienced hands and following dilatation of the pupils, is not an adequate means of excluding early retinopathy. The gold standard technique is digital retinal photography of both eyes following dilatation, and examination of the images by an experienced professional who analyses such images regularly (Figure 11.5). Dilatation should be achieved using a short-acting topical mydriatic such as tropicamide 0.5%. Retinopathy is present at the time of diagnosis in 37% of type 2 patients, and newly diagnosed individuals should not be left to wait 12 months before the annual screen is organised.

Urinary microalbumin screening

Dipstix are available for the detection of microalbumin, but for accurate quantification a laboratory will measure the albumin: creatinine ratio. This is abnormal if >2.5 for men and >3.5 for women. A positive finding should be followed up with a second sample as spurious positive results may occur, particularly if infection is present. If unconfirmed on a second sample then a third should be arranged, and two out of three positive is considered conclusive. Angiotensin converting enzyme inhibitors (ACEI) and tight control of blood pressure in patients with urinary microalbumin are extremely beneficial (see Chapter 12).

Figure 11.5 A digital retinal photograph showing extensive background and macular changes (with thanks to Dr Paul O'Hare).

Depression screening

As with many long-term health problems, patients with diabetes are at significantly higher risk of depression, and symptoms may not be reported. Active questioning to screen for depressive symptoms should be part of an annual diabetes review. In the UK, this involves the use of two validated screening questions. Positive indications of an underlying depression should be followed by a formal assessment using a validated instrument such as the PHQ-9 (see Chapter 16).

Other issues that need to be addressed on a regular basis include:

- **Erectile dysfunction:** Unless clearly inappropriate a question about erectile dysfunction should be included in an annual review to male patients. This problem is common and treatable, but may go unreported because of embarrassment. If medication is required (e.g. Sildenafil) this should be placed in the 'Repeats' screen along with other medication unless there is a reason not to.
- **Driving safety:** In the UK, patients treated with oral medication should be advised to inform the Driving and Vehicle Licensing Authority (DVLA), even though currently this is not legally required unless they have a complication likely to impair driving ability (e.g. visual or affecting limb function). Provided they satisfy this criterion they will be able to retain their 'til 70' licence but given information about when and how to inform DVLA of changes in circumstances. If they do not inform the DVLA they will not have actually broken the law, but if in future they then do develop problems affecting driving ability they may not realise that they then are obliged to report them. They are on stronger grounds regarding insurance if they have informed the DVLA and received this advice. Patients on insulin should all be advised that they are legally obliged to inform the DVLA and this advice should be written in the notes. They are likely to be allowed to continue driving provided they have adequate glycaemic control, are free of disabling hypoglycaemia, have hypoglycaemia awareness, and no complications that affect driving ability. The DVLA guidelines are updated every 6 months so if in doubt it is worth accessing their website (given below).
- **A holistic perspective:** It is easy to become fixated on 'box-ticking' when conducting surveillance reviews. Box-ticking is, in fact, extremely important if an assessment is to be comprehensive, and screen templates may facilitate this process. But an assessment should also include some protected time for the 'free-text' issues that are important for quality of life. This is, after all, one of the major goals of diabetes management. These aspects are not as easily quantified or measured but are valued by patients. Relationship issues, educational progress, family support, work stress and other anxieties, and future life plans may all come to light to a receptive ear in a supportive environment. Spending time on these will build the clinician-patient relationship and reap benefits in future when difficult management decisions need to be shared.

Summary

Surveillance for complications is a major component of diabetes care, and should take the form of regular reviews (at least annually) with protected time for a comprehensive assessment of the patient's needs. It cannot be managed by a single health care professional, but requires a teamwork approach using a shared care protocol, adapted to locally available resources and understood by all involved. This protocol should, where possible, be discussed with the patient to facilitate the early detection and treatment of complications. Routine surveillance should also include an exploration of the psycho-social issues that affect quality of life but that may not otherwise be reported.

Further reading

Driving and Vehicle Licensing Authority. *'At a Glance' Guide to Medical Standards of Fitness to Drive*. www.dvla.gov.uk/medical/ataglance.aspx
National Institute for Health and Clinical Excellence. *Clinical Guideline 66. Diabetes – type 2 (update)*. May 2008.

CHAPTER 12

Kidney Disease in Diabetes

Tim Holt[1] and Sudhesh Kumar[2]

[1]Health Sciences Research Institute, Warwick Medical School, University of Warwick, Coventry, UK
[2]Clinical Sciences Research Institute, Warwick Medical School, University of Warwick; and WISDEM, University Hospital, Coventry, UK

OVERVIEW

- Nephropathy may already be established at presentation in type 2 patients and is a common long-term complication for those with type 1 diabetes

- An increasing proportion of patients are living long enough to develop end stage renal failure, requiring expansion of renal replacement services

- Progression of renal impairment is reduced through control of blood pressure, glycaemia and lipids, and angiotensin converting enzyme inhibition

- Angiotensin converting enzyme inhibitors should be offered to all patients with any degree of albuminuria unless contraindicated

- Monitoring of renal function is an important task for primary care, and thresholds for referral to secondary care should be locally agreed and widely understood

- Renal impairment affects other aspects of diabetes management including choice of drugs and dosages

Introduction

Despite improvements in early detection, prevention, and treatment, diabetic nephropathy is still a major cause of mortality and morbidity. At 25 years from diagnosis of diabetes, around one-third of type 1 patients and a fifth of those with type 2 have end stage renal failure, although these figures are improving. The development of proteinuria is usually the first indication. Worsening renal function makes associated hypertension more difficult to control, leading to more generalised vascular disease and further renal damage. Untreated, renal function may deteriorate to the point of dialysis dependence typically over a period of years.

Looking on the brighter side, urinalysis detects at an early stage a problem whose natural history can now be modified, and where this is not possible or unsuccessful, adequate quality of life can usually be maintained through dialysis or transplantation. Mortality rates in dialysis and transplant patients are falling. Urinary albumin can now be detected at concentrations lower than that possible through conventional urinalysis. As discussed below, this 'microalbumin' signals the need for active measures to control risk factors and prevent further progression.

Epidemiology

Diabetic nephropathy is the most common specific primary renal diagnosis in patients entering UK programmes for renal replacement therapy (RRT), accounting for around 22% of new cases in 2006. The ratio of men to women is 1.6, due to accompanying renovascular disease which is commoner in men. The prevalence in the population is increasing, reflecting the rising prevalence of diabetes, improved survival and treatment, and a rise in referral rates for RRT particularly in the type 2 population, with better access to dialysis units.

Van Dijk and colleagues describe the variation across different European centres (Van Dijk *et al.* 2005). Their figures show a steady rise in incidence of RRT throughout the 1990s, particularly among type 2 patients, where an increase of nearly 12% per year was observed (Figure 12.1). In the older age groups the ratio of men to women increased during this decade. Improved mortality rates from cardiovascular disease may partly explain this trend. Whilst survival rates for dialysis patients are generally improving, mortality among those with diabetic nephropathy is still higher than in those with other causes of renal disease, partly due to co-morbidity including cardiovascular disease.

The cyclical nature of causation in diabetic nephropathy (Boxes 12.1 and 12.2) makes it extremely worthwhile as a preventive endeavour, because the benefits (e.g. of blood pressure control) feed back on themselves in the long run.

Box 12.1 **Breaking the cycle**

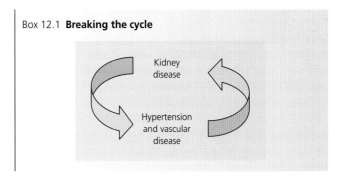

ABC of Diabetes, 6th edition. By T. Holt and S. Kumar.
Published 2010 by Blackwell Publishing.

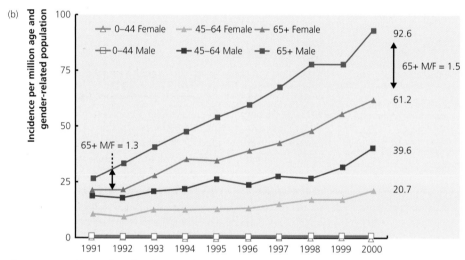

Figure 12.1 Incidence of renal replacement therapy (RRT) is relatively stable for type 1 patients (a) compared with type 2 populations (b), where needs are escalating, particularly in older men. Reproduced with permission from Van Dijk *et al. Kidney International* 2005;**67**:1489–99.

Pathological mechanisms in diabetic nephropathy are complex, and involve genetic factors as well as glycaemia, lipids, smoking and blood pressure. Microvascular and macrovascular factors conspire in the progression of this complication, a cycle reinforced by secondary hypertension

---

Box 12.2 Factors promoting the development and progression of nephropathy

- Blood pressure
- Poor glycaemic control
- Dyslipidaemia
- Smoking
- High protein intake
- Small kidneys
- Genetic factors

Clinical presentation

Type 1 patients rarely develop signs of nephropathy prior to 5 years following diagnosis of diabetes. They typically have normal blood pressure and renal function at presentation. Type 2 patients have often had diabetes for several years before diagnosis and a proportion have established nephropathy from the start. Many have co-existing hypertension and may be already at the stage of impaired renal function. Diabetic nephropathy can affect any patient but is commoner in those of Afro-Caribbean and South Asian ethnicities.

The stages of diabetic nephropathy
See Table 12.1.

Decline in glomerular filtration rate (GFR)
The estimated GFR is a measure of creatinine clearance, and progressively declines in patients with established diabetic nephropathy. However, as Table 12.1 indicates, prior to this decline the

Table 12.1 Stages of progression of diabetic nephropathy.

	Normal (I)	Incipient (II)	Persistent (III)	Clinical (IV)	End stage (V)
Albuminuria (mg/24 h)	<20	20–300 (microalbuminuria)	≥300 (up to 15 g/day)	≥300 (up to 15 g/day)	≥300 (can fall)
Glomerular filtration rate (ml/min)	High/normal Hyperfiltration	Normal/high	Normal or decreased	Decreased	Greatly decreased
Serum creatinine (μmol/l)	Normal 60–100	Normal 60–120	High normal 80–120	High 120–400	Very high >400
Blood pressure (mm Hg)	Normal	Slightly increased	Increased	Increased	Increased
Clinical signs	None	None	Anaemia ± oedema, increased blood pressure, may be none	Anaemia ± oedema, increased blood pressure, may be none	Anaemia ± oedema, increased blood pressure, uraemic symptoms

GFR may in fact be high. This generally applies at the stage of microalbuminuria (stage II) but also at the earlier stage I, which is not associated with any other abnormal investigation findings. This asymptomatic 'hyperfiltration' phase may or may not progress to the later stages depending on how successfully blood pressure and other factors are controlled. Stage I individuals are not readily identifiable in clinical practice, but this should encourage clinicians to offer tight control of these risk factors to everyone with diabetes, all of whom are potentially at risk of nephropathy.

How will the patient feel?

The early stages of nephropathy are asymptomatic, which is one reason why screening is so important. Gradually, blood pressure may become more difficult to control, normocytic anaemia occurs, peripheral oedema may be evident, and the malaise and nausea of uraemia develop (Box 12.3). As renal function declines further, the symptoms related to uraemia and anaemia become progressively worse and at this stage the patient is entering an 'end stage' where the need for dialysis is impending.

Box 12.3 **Signs and symptoms of uraemia**

Malaise	Nocturia
Pallor	Dyspnoea
Hiccoughs	Oedema
Nausea	Confusion
Pruritis	Pericarditis

Microalbuminuria

Renal damage is typically gradual and progressive, so the earlier it is detected the better. Before the onset of proteinuria (in which albumin is detectable at a concentration of >200 mg/l), milder degrees may be present that will be missed by conventional urinalysis. Detection of protein in the urine is more meaningful if it is measured as a ratio of urinary albumin to creatinine concentrations, or as a 24-hour excretion rate.

Microalbuminuria is defined as an albumin excretion rate of 30–300 mg/24 hours, or an albumin: creatinine ratio of >2.5 mg/mmol/l (for men) and >3.5 mg/mmol/l (for women) (Table 12.2). Stix are now available that can detect both microalbumin and creatinine to estimate this ratio. The first morning sample after rising is preferable to samples taken later in the day. Regular

Table 12.2 Diagnostic definitions of microalbuminuria and proteinuria. An albumin creatinine ratio of 30 mg/mmol is approximately equivalent to a protein creatinine ratio of 50 mg/mmol.

	Urinary albumin concentration (mg/l)	Albumin: creatinine ratio	24-hour albumin excretion (mg/24 hr)
Normal	<20	<2.5 (men) <3.5 (women)	<30
Microalbuminuria	20–200	>2.5 (men) >3.5 (women)	30–300
Proteinuria	>200	>30	>300

urinalysis for microalbumin should be part of routine surveillance in diabetes, but a positive finding must be repeated to confirm, and infection excluded as well. A sample should then be sent to the laboratory to measure the ratio more accurately, or alternatively a 24-hour urine collection for albumin can be arranged.

Investigation of suspected nephropathy

Nephropathy is a well recognised and not uncommon complication in diabetes, usually starting with albuminuria that progresses over time. However, other causes of kidney disease might affect someone with diabetes, and there are many potential causes of proteinuria. So the initial question is whether the diagnosis can be made based on the clinical presentation, or whether further investigations including renal biopsy are justified.

Patients with diabetes who develop microalbumin and who are detected through routine surveillance will not need invasive investigations at this stage. They should have a midstream specimen of urine (MSU) taken to exclude infection, and provided this is sterile and acellular it is safe to continue follow-up on the assumption that they have stage II (incipient) nephropathy (see Table 12.1).

Those with actual proteinuria (detectable on conventional urinalysis suggesting a urinary albumin concentration >200 mg/l) should similarly have infection, pyuria and haematuria excluded through MSU. It may be worth measuring albumin excretion through a 24-hour urine collection, to provide a baseline for future progression. Such patients should also have an ultrasound examination of the renal tract, to support the clinical examination in excluding unexpected pathology such as a tumour. For those with renal impairment, ultrasound also helps to exclude obstructive causes, particularly in men, who may have prostatic enlargement, or in either sex as a result of autonomic neuropathy causing chronic urinary retention (Box 12.4).

A blood test for C-reactive protein and antinuclear factor is worthwhile in patients with proteinuria. Routine biochemistry should reveal normal serum albumin levels. A patient with low albumin levels and oedema (nephrotic syndrome) is likely to have a different cause for their proteinuria (see Box 12.4). If the cause is diabetic nephropathy, at the point where proteinuria becomes detectable on conventional stix, it is likely that the e-GFR will be at least borderline, if not actually abnormal.

> **Box 12.4 Abrupt onset of proteinuria is never due to diabetes**
>
> Patients not following the typical pattern of presentation may have another cause of renal disease that might benefit from other types of treatment. Other causes are more likely to affect type 2 patients, as they tend to be commoner with increasing age

Patients with proteinuria due to diabetic nephropathy usually also have retinopathy. If this is not present then other causes of renal disease need considering (Box 12.5).

Anaemia occurs relatively early in diabetic nephropathy compared with other causes of kidney disease, so it is not unusual for this anaemia to be symptomatic at the point where the urea and creatinine are not particularly high.

Patients with renal artery stenosis may be identified if a decline in renal function (sometimes dramatic) occurs after commencing ACE inhibitors. A vascular bruit may be evident on auscultating the abdomen. Such patients should be referred for imaging of the renal arteries and may benefit from interventions to improve renovascular function including angioplasty.

> **Box 12.5 Who needs other investigations?**
>
> • Type 1 patients developing proteinuria without having been through a microalbuminuria stage
> • Pyuria or haematuria on MSU
> • Family history of other renal disease
> • Absence of retinopathy
> • Nephrotic syndrome
> • Features of nephritis: haematuria, raised C-reactive protein
> • Those showing an abrupt decline in renal function following ACE inhibition

Histological features of diabetic nephropathy

Renal biopsy

Renal biopsy is carried out via a posterior approach through the lumbar musculature, under local anaesthetic, and guided by ultrasound. In preparation, patients should have clotting function and platelet count checked, and be fasted for 6 hours. Macroscopic haematuria frequently occurs after this procedure, and is almost always self-limiting.

Figure 12.2 Diabetic glomerulosclerosis with Kimmelstiel-Wilson nodules.

Histology

The typical histological signs of diabetic nephropathy are diabetic glomerulosclerosis with mesangial expansion and thickening of the basement membrane. The classical features evident in the later stages are Kimmelstiel-Wilson nodules, associated with hyalinisation of the efferent and afferent arterioles (Figure 12.2).

Primary prevention

Diabetic nephropathy is essentially a microvascular complication, but as indicated above, it may trigger macrovascular processes as well that promote its further progression. This 'vicious cycle' should encourage not only early intervention but also prevention if possible. The most effective means of achieving this are through:

• Glycaemic control
• Blood pressure control
• Smoking cessation

These should be offered to all patients with diabetes, but treatment targets should be tightened when the early stages of nephropathy develop. In patients with no current signs of nephropathy, targets need to be balanced against other issues including quality of life and risks of over-treatment. This particularly applies to elderly patients and those whose life-expectancy is already limited.

Treatment of diabetic nephropathy

The patient with established nephropathy is not only at risk of end stage renal failure but also of cardiovascular complications including myocardial infarction. A high proportion of patients with proteinuria have co-existing coronary artery disease, which may be asymptomatic. It is also likely that other microvascular disease is present, and almost all have co-existing retinopathy.

Secondary prevention

The mainstay of treatment of diabetic nephropathy is secondary prevention through tight blood pressure and glycaemic control, lipid management and smoking cessation if appropriate (Box 12.6). Patients entering the symptomatic stage should be referred and managed by a nephrologist in addition to any follow-up occurring in primary care. Good communication between primary and secondary care is important to achieve the best outcomes and the best use of specialist expertise.

Box 12.6 Treatment targets in diabetic nephropathy

Treatment targets in diabetic nephropathy should be individually tailored, but generally aim for:

Blood pressure <130/80
HbA1c <6.5% (48 mmol/mol)
Total cholesterol <4.0 mmol/l and LDL <2.0 mmol/l
Non-smoker status

In established nephropathy with proteinuria, it is safe to assume the patient has widespread microvascular and macrovascular (including coronary artery) disease

---

Angiotensin converting enzyme inhibitors (ACEIs)

Angiotensin converting enzyme inhibitors (Box 12.7) have been shown to reduce progression of diabetic nephropathy, and should be offered to all patients with any degree of albuminuria, even if the blood pressure is normal. They reduce the risk of end stage renal failure requiring dialysis or transplantation, and improve all-cause mortality. Patients may fail to tolerate ACEIs for a number of reasons. Cough is a relatively common side effect and requires substitution of the drug with an angiotensin 2 receptor blocker. These drugs have also been shown to reduce progression to end stage renal failure, but not all-cause mortality, and ACEIs are still the preferred option if tolerated (Box 12.8).

Box 12.7 Currently available Angiotensin converting enzyme inhibitors (ACEIs) and Angiotensin 2 receptor blockers

ACEIs	Angiotensin 2 receptor blockers
Ramipril	Candesartan
Lisinopril	Valsartan
Enalapril	Losartan
Captopril	Irbesartan
Trandolapril	Telmisartan
Quinapril	Eprosartan
Perindopril	Olmesartan
Cilazapril	
Fosinopril	
Moexipril	

Box 12.8 Every effort should be made to help the patient tolerate ACEI or A2RB

ACE inhibition is a vital component of the secondary prevention of diabetic nephropathy. All too often, ACEIs are withdrawn due to minor side effects without considering other management options, denying the patient the opportunity to benefit in the long term from this therapy. Sometimes the patient does not appreciate the

---

potential benefits and too readily opts for other means of blood pressure control.

If cough occurs with ACEI offer an A2RB, which will not cause cough.

If other side effects occur, review the schedule and adjust other medication accordingly:

Dizziness. Is the patient also taking diuretics? Do they really need them at this dose? Are they fluid depleted? Even though the symptom may have been precipitated by the addition of ACEI, it may be resolved by withdrawal of other drugs such as a thiazide or a beta blocker instead of the ACEI. Angiotensin converting enzyme inhibitors sometimes produce a 'first dose hypotension' effect, but, provided renal function has not deteriorated, it may be safe to continue by giving the drug before bed unless the patient is at risk of night-time falls. Clearly, this advice needs to be tailored to the individual. Start at the lowest possible dose and titrate upwards, monitoring blood pressure and renal function.

Deterioration in renal function. Consider withdrawal of diuretics prior to commencing ACE inhibition, and check blood pressure and renal function before and soon after starting therapy and after each dose increase. If a decline in e-GFR occurs, consider other drugs that may be contributing, such as Non-steroidal anti-inflammatory drugs (NSAIDs) and review the need for them rather than withdrawing the ACEI unless this is really necessary.

Even a small dose of ACEI is better than nothing.

For those who really cannot tolerate ACEIs, tight blood pressure control with other agents is still a priority

Lipid management and aspirin

Patients with established proteinuria due to diabetic nephropathy are at high risk of cardiovascular events and justify the same approach to cardiovascular risk reduction as those with known coronary artery disease. In addition to lipid-lowering agents (which are recommended anyway for most people with diabetes) this includes aspirin in a high proportion of patients, particularly those with established CVD. Aspirin sometimes has an adverse effect on renal function but at low dose the benefits generally outweigh this risk provided GFR is greater than 15 ml/min.

Protein restriction

There is a role for protein restriction in diabetic nephropathy but this is generally recommended only if intake is excessive. Orally ingested protein increases urea production and places a strain on the kidneys, exacerbating uraemia in the later, symptomatic stages. At earlier stages there is some evidence that protein restriction reduces the decline in GFR, but this effect is minor, and restriction is not recommended unless the protein intake is particularly high. Assessment by a dietician working in collaboration with the nephrologist is useful to clarify this in each individual case.

Referral to secondary care

Early nephropathy is likely to be identified in primary care, and for much of the course of the disease management based in primary care is appropriate, to maintain tight control of blood pressure (with ACEIs or A2RB), blood glucose and lipids. Liaison with secondary care is important, as well as clearly understood thresholds for referral to a nephrologist. Secondary care expertise is important at the stages where the patient has become symptomatic and particularly as they progress towards dialysis dependence and develop further nephrological complications including secondary hyperparathyroidism with osteomalacia. Access to secondary care varies depending on the health care infrastructure available. In the UK, it is usual to refer patients whose e-GFR has fallen below 25 ml/min, those with symptoms of uraemia, or those with other complications.

Other problems

Acute

Patients with established nephropathy may develop acute problems that require prompt action. Practitioners caring for such patients must be aware of the necessary action required. The detailed management of these is beyond the scope of this book, but we include here some important examples.

Hyperkalaemia. Potassium levels are prone to rise with declining renal function, and are liable to rise further in response to ACEI or A2RBs. Such patients require close monitoring. Levels rising above 5.7 mmol/l require prompt action and those above 6 mmol/l are an emergency due to risk of fatal arrhythmias.

Acute deterioration in renal function. This may occur for a number of reasons and is more likely in a patient with already compromised renal function. Causes may be pre-renal (e.g. dehydration or shock from any cause), renal (including drug therapy, sepsis, myoglobinaemia), or post-renal (e.g. obstruction due to retention or by tumour). The patient should be transferred urgently to secondary care, their hydration status assessed, precipitating factors identified, and the need for urgent dialysis or other support determined.

Overwhelming infection. Patients with diabetic nephropathy are at higher risk from ascending urinary infection, which may cause not only an acute pyelonephritis and septicaemia, but also an acute papillary necrosis with further decline in renal function. Urinary infection must be actively managed and if there is evidence of involvement of the kidneys this should be undertaken in hospital with intravenous antibiotics.

More gradual

More gradual decline in renal function may occur in patients taking over-the-counter NSAIDs without their clinician's awareness, and occasionally patients taking statins may develop a low grade myositis, which is not reported but causes renal impairment due to undetected myoglobinaemia.

Secondary hyperparathyroidism is a complication of renal failure of any cause, and puts the patient at risk of osteomalacia and pathological fractures.

Erythropoietin deficiency

The normocytic anaemia associated with renal failure is caused partly by deficiency of the hormone erythropoietin (EPO), which

is produced by the kidney and promotes erythrocyte production in the bone marrow. This anaemia tends to occur earlier in the course of nephropathy in diabetes than it does in other forms of renal disease. Treatment with replacement EPO injections is extremely effective and can greatly improve quality of life. Other factors contributing to the anaemia such as iron or folate deficiency should be excluded prior to starting therapy (Box 12.9).

Box 12.9 **Treatment of diabetic nephropathy**

Tight blood pressure control with ACEIs or A2RBs
Tight glycaemic control
Smoking cessation
Control of hyperlipidaemia if present
Protein restriction if intake excessive in the earlier stages, and for symptom relief later on
Erythropoietin for anaemia
Haemodialysis or continuous ambulatory peritoneal dialysis
Renal transplantation

Prescribing issues in people with renal impairment

Numerous drugs must be used with caution in people with kidney disease, and some of these are particularly relevant to those with diabetes. They include drugs liable to worsen renal function, and those in which the renal impairment may make the drug unsafe. Some of these are described below, but this list is not comprehensive and only includes drugs particularly relevant to diabetes care. If in doubt consult a formulary before prescribing any new drug to a patient with renal impairment.

Angiotensin converting enzyme inhibitors (ACEIs). These drugs are an important (in fact central) component of the treatment of diabetic nephropathy, and in the long run should improve renal outcomes. However, in some cases renal function may decline, particularly after the drug is first started, and this should always be done with close monitoring of renal function. A patient whose renal function deteriorates rapidly after the introduction of ACEI might have renal artery stenosis, and may require investigation to exclude this. As mentioned above, it may be worth withdrawing other drugs such as NSAIDs in order to ensure that the patient tolerates the ACEI and thereby benefits from its long-term reno-protective effect.

Beta blockers. Certain beta blockers are excreted through the urine and lower doses will be required. These include atenolol, nebivolol, celiprolol, acebutalol and sotalol.

Bezafibrate and gemfibrozil are similarly affected and lower starting doses are appropriate. Bezafibrate should not be given if the creatinine clearance is less than 15 ml/min and gemfibrozil if less than 30 ml/min.

Calcium channel blockers (CCBs). Some CCBs are affected by renal impairment and doses may need to be adjusted accordingly, or in some cases the drug avoided. Amlodipine and felodipine are unaffected.

Escitalopram, fluvoxamine and paroxetine. Depression is common in diabetes (see page 75), particularly where other chronic conditions such as renal failure are present, and antidepressants are likely to be offered to such patients. Many are safe, but the formulary should be consulted and some such as escitalopram, fluvoxamine and paroxetine carry cautions.

Insulin metabolism is affected by severe renal impairment and this may require dose reductions as renal failure progresses.

Metformin is the only biguanide currently licensed for the treatment of diabetes. One of its adverse effects is lactic acidosis, and this is much more likely to occur in people with renal impairment. Past recommendations have been to avoid metformin in patients with a serum creatinine >150 mcmol/l. Converting this advice to an e-GFR level is difficult as it depends on age and sex, but generally a GFR level of 30 ml/min is appropriate, below which metformin should not be prescribed. A patient may have been taking metformin for a long time, but as renal function declines this level may be reached and the drug should then be withdrawn and others used instead.

Nitrates should be used with caution in severe renal impairment.

Non-steroidal anti-inflammatory drugs (NSAIDs). Whilst not specific to diabetes care these are commonly used drugs that may impair renal function, and should be avoided if impairment is moderate or severe. If mild, these drugs may be used at the lowest effective dose and with close monitoring of renal function. These side effects are more likely if co-administered with ACEIs, and this interaction may mean that the patient is denied the benefits of ACEIs to preserve renal function.

Rosiglitazone should be used with caution if the creatinine clearance is less than 30 ml/min.

Statins. Most patients with diabetes should be prescribed statins, and this particularly includes those with nephropathy, where control of lipid levels is a priority. Simvastatin, rosuvastatin and pravastatin are renally excreted, requiring lower doses, and atorvastatin may be a safer option depending on the level of renal function.

Sulphonylureas. Some sulphonylureas are eliminated largely by the kidney, including glibenclamide and tolbutamide. Renal impairment will lead to prolonged duration of their effects, with risk of hypoglycaemia. Shorter acting agents including gliclazide are now in more common use, and are largely metabolised without requiring renal clearance. Their use in patients with nephropathy is preferable, although doses may still need to be lowered.

Thiazide diuretics are relatively ineffective as diuretics if creatinine clearance is less that 30 ml/min. As antihypertensive drugs they are not contraindicated in diabetes but other options may be preferable to avoid aggravating hyperglycaemia and the hyperuricaemia associated with renal impairment.

Varenicline is a new drug prescribed to assist with smoking cessation, another important treatment of diabetic nephropathy. If creatinine clearance is less than 30 ml/min then doses should be adjusted according to the manufacturers instructions.

Summary

The global rise in diabetes prevalence and improvements in cardiovascular mortality are increasing the need for renal replacement therapy across the world, as rising numbers of patients (particularly type 2) survive to the end stage of renal failure. This trend will inevitably continue, requiring an expansion of the availability of dialysis and renal transplantation services. Programmes to prevent progression to the later stages of diabetic nephropathy are essential and should be part of the organisational infrastructure of all primary care teams. Liaison between primary and secondary care and clear referral pathways are important to promote optimal outcomes and make the best use of specialist expertise.

Further reading

Farrington K, Udayaraj U, Gilg J, Feest T, Feehally J. New adult patients starting renal replacement therapy in the UK in 2006. In: *UK Renal Registry Report* (Ansell D, Feehally J, Feest TG, Tomson C, Williams AJ, Warwick G, eds). UK Renal Registry, Bristol, 2007.

NICE Guidance. http://guidance.nice.org.uk/F.

SIGN Guidance. http://www.sign.ac.uk/pdf/sign103.pdf.

Van Dijk KJ, Jager B, Stengel C, Renal replacement therapy for diabetic end-stage renal disease: Data from 10 registries in Europe (1991–2000). *Kidney Int* 2005;**67**:1489–99.

CHAPTER 13

Eye Disease in Diabetes

Tim Holt[1] and Sudhesh Kumar[2]

[1] Health Sciences Research Institute, Warwick Medical School, University of Warwick, Coventry, UK
[2] Clinical Sciences Research Institute, Warwick Medical School, University of Warwick; and WISDEM, University Hospital, Coventry, UK

OVERVIEW

- Diabetic retinopathy is still the leading cause of blindness in those under 65 years in industrialised countries

- Early detection enables effective interventions to prevent visual loss

- Screening for retinopathy should be available to all adult patients with diabetes

- Screening programmes require effective coordination between primary care services, diabetologists and ophthalmologists

- Patients with any degree of retinopathy require tight control of vascular risk factors

- Other eye problems in diabetes include glaucoma, cataract, optic neuropathy and ocular palsies

Introduction

Diabetic retinopathy is common, serious and costly, detectable in a pre-symptomatic phase, and treatable with widely available and effective interventions to prevent progression to disabling visual loss. Screening for retinopathy is therefore a priority area of diabetes care. Loss of vision is perhaps the complication patients fear the most, and despite improving figures this is still the commonest cause of blindness in working age people in industrialised countries.

Modern ophthalmologic techniques including laser therapy, commencing in the 1970s have perhaps been the single most significant advance in the management of diabetes since the discovery of insulin. Widespread use of laser followed the US Diabetes Retinopathy Study (DRS), which first demonstrated its effectiveness in 1974.

Patients newly diagnosed with diabetes should be told about all the possible complications of their condition. In the case of retinopathy there is a good chance that control of risk factors combined with regular surveillance and early treatment of problems will prevent future disability.

Screening techniques

As discussed in the surveillance chapter, all adult patients with diabetes should be offered retinopathy screening at diagnosis and

ABC of Diabetes, 6th edition. By T. Holt and S. Kumar.
Published 2010 by Blackwell Publishing.

annually thereafter. This involves bilateral digital photography of both fundi following pupillary dilatation. A short-acting topical mydriatic such as tropicamide 0.5% is usually used. A possible contra-indication is a history of acute angle-closure glaucoma and caution should be applied in those with risk factors for this condition (older, hypermetropic patients) but serious problems are uncommon. Transient stinging of the eyes is to be expected but is not serious. Visual acuity should be measured in both eyes prior to dilatation.

Early detection of changes (described below) should then be followed up through further assessment, more frequent review and treatment where indicated.

Pathogenesis

Diabetic retinopathy is largely a microvascular complication, involving disease in the small vessels particularly of the basement membrane. Damage to these vessels results in increased permeability and leakage of blood or plasma into the extravascular space, with secondary thickening of the basement membrane. Disruption of the blood supply causes localised tissue hypoxia, triggering release of vascular growth factors. It is these that promote the proliferation of new vessels during the later stages in both the retina and vitreous humour. Vascular insufficiency due to atheroma of the larger vessels supplying the eye, or micro-emboli from carotid artery disease may further reduce tissue perfusion and oxygenation. Exudation and haemorrhage lead to fibrosis, further damaging visual function and predisposing to retinal detachment.

Background retinopathy

Risk of retinopathy correlates strongly with the duration of diabetes. Background changes are almost universal after 20 years of type 1 diabetes, and are frequently present at diagnosis in type 2 patients (Figure 13.1). The hallmark lesions are *microaneurysms*, which are visible on fundoscopy as minute 'dot' haemorrhages. Microaneurysms are not actually haemorrhages but are localised dilatations of capillaries. The small vessels themselves are typically too small to be detected, which results in the impression of an isolated haemorrhage. In contrast, 'blot' haemorrhages are indeed due to leakage of blood, usually into the nerve fibres above the

Figure 13.1 Background retinopathy with a few microaneurysms only. This stage is not likely to threaten vision in the near future but tight control of vascular risk factors is important to reduce progression (photograph courtsey of Dr Sailesh Sankar, consultant Physician, University Hospital, Coventry).

Figure 13.3 The same eye as in Fig 13.2, showing relative sparing of the macular region, but the retina is generally ischaemic and at risk of progression to sight threatening neovascularisation (photograph courtsey of Dr Sailesh Sankar, Consultant Physician, University Hospital, Coventry).

basement membrane. They are noticeably larger and often irregular in outline.

Background changes do not cause visual loss but do signify significant vascular disease and, particularly when occurring close to the visual axis, may require more frequent screening examinations.

Pre-proliferative retinopathy

Cotton wool spots

Localised ischaemia due to closure of diseased blood vessels results in a 'cotton wool' appearance (Figures 13.2 and 13.3), previously referred to as 'soft exudates', which is a misnomer as the process does not actually involve leakage or exudation. Such changes do not

usually affect acuity themselves, but may herald the development of neovascularisation.

Hard exudates

Leakage of lipids from damaged capillaries leads to 'hard exudates', which, although not involving neovascularisation, may result in permanent visual loss through damage to the macula and fovea.

Venous beading and **intra-retinal microvascular abnormalities** (IRMAs) are further signs of pre-proliferative retinopathy.

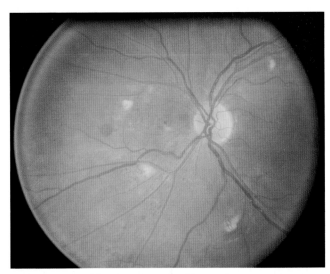

Figure 13.2 Pre-proliferative retinopathy with several cotton wool spots as well as background microaneurysms and blot haemorrhages (photograph courtsey of Dr Sailesh Sankar, Consultant Physician, University Hospital, Coventry).

Figure 13.4 Maculopathy in a patient with established background changes, indicated by microaneurysms and blot haemorrhages (photograph courtsey of Dr Sailesh Sankar, Consultant Physician, University Hospital, Coventry).

Figure 13.5 Pre-proliferative diabetic retinopathy with exudative maculopathy. At least two cotton wool spots indicate retinal ischaemia. There are multiple microaneurysms and haemorrhages, venous beading, and both linear and stellate exudates at the macula, with arterio-venous nipping due to coexisting hypertension (photograph courtsey of Dr Paul O'Hare and Dr Vinod Patel, Warwick Medical School).

Figure 13.6 Proliferative diabetic retinopathy showing new vessel formation and vitreous haemorrhages (photograph courtsey of Dr Sailesh Sankar, consultant Physician, University Hospital, Coventry).

Diabetic maculopathy

Increased permeability of the retinal vessels may result in localised oedema, even in the absence of exudates or new vessels (Figure 13.4). When this occurs at the macula it can result in a very acute deterioration in acuity over a period of hours. This complication is difficult to foresee but is treatable, so patients should be aware of the need to report changes in acuity even if a recent screening examination was satisfactory. Exudative maculopathy may occur in a patient with more advanced pre-proliferative disease (Figure 13.5).

Proliferative retinopathy

The more serious forms of diabetic retinopathy, associated with permanent visual loss, are usually the result of failure of preventive interventions allowing proliferative changes involving new vessel growth (Figure 13.6).

Neovascularisation

Figure 13.7 shows the typical appearance of new vessel formation. These develop in response to vascular growth factors released in response to tissue hypoxia in the basement membrane. In contrast to macular oedema, these changes usually develop gradually and progressively, providing opportunities for prevention. It is unusual for neovascularisation to develop without a recognisable pre-proliferative phase. If preventive measures fail, neovascularisation may result in permanent loss of acuity or visual field.

Sequelae of new vessel growth

New vessels usually arise of the venous side of the circulation and are not normal vessels – they are friable and bleed easily, resulting

Figure 13.7 New vessels in the peripheral retina, with exudates (photograph courtsey of Dr Sailesh Sankar, consultant Physician, University Hospital, Coventry).

in vitreous haemorrhage and irreversible fibrosis of the surrounding tissues (Figure 13.8). This fibrosis causes traction on the underlying retina, promoting retinal detachment with accumulation of fluid between the neural and pigmented layers.

Further assessment of established retinopathy

Microaneurysms are commonly detected on screening examinations and usually require no immediate action other than attention to risk factors, particularly glycaemic control. Patients should be

Figure 13.8 Extensive haemorrhage into the subhyaloid layer between the retina and the vitreous humour resulting from proliferative retinopathy (photograph courtsey of Dr Sailesh Sankar, consultant Physician, University Hospital, Coventry).

aware of the importance of attending future examinations, but unless the background changes are close to the macula, annual follow-up will probably be appropriate. Pre-proliferative changes, particularly when close to the visual axis, require further assessment with an ophthalmologist, preferably one with an interest in diabetic eye disease.

In addition to slit lamp examination and retinal photography, a number of techniques are used to further evaluate the eye in diabetes.

Fluorescein angiography may be used to highlight small vessels that are otherwise too small to see. This helps in the assessment of the microcirculation, and can distinguish (for instance) between generalised venous dilatation and venous beading, the latter much more significant prognostically and associated with closure of the surrounding capillary circulation. It helps to distinguish new vessels from normal vessels. The latter typically form a branching pattern like a tree, whilst abnormal new vessels frequently join up with themselves again to form arcs or networks of vessels called 'rete'. Fluoroscein angiography can also distinguish cotton wool spots (which are ischaemic areas of underperfusion) from areas associated with haemorrhage and exudation.

Ocular coherence tomography may be useful to determine the presence of traction on the macula in a patient with maculopathy (Figure 13.9), as this condition also involves oedema and the relative contribution of each is not always evident on slit lamp examination or photography.

Measurement of intra-ocular pressure is important in the assessment of anyone with established retinopathy, particularly those with proliferative retinopathy. Peripheral new vessels may be missed on screening examinations and are often associated with rubeosis iridis, predisposing to secondary glaucoma (see below).

Treatment options

Treatment of retinopathy depends largely on the stage of the disease, but also on other factors, including the location. A distinction is made between new vessels at the disc (NVD) and new vessels elsewhere (NVE).

Pre-proliferative changes usually only require tightening control of vascular risk factors, although maculopathy may require laser treatment localised to the macula to reduce leakage from blood vessels.

Pan-retinal photocoagulation

Proliferative retinopathy is caused by the release of vascular growth factors from ischaemic retinal tissue. Laser treatment destroys the upper layer to reduce the oxygen requirement of the ischaemic retina, and thereby reduces the release of the factors that promote new vessel growth. For this to be effective, between 1000 and 2000 separate 'burns' may be required during a treatment course and these are distributed all over the retina, particularly the peripheral areas (also known as 'scatter laser therapy'). This may reduce peripheral vision, but is necessary to preserve the function of the visual axis (Figure 13.10). This treatment is not only effective at reducing visual loss but may also eventually improve acuity where this is reduced.

Vitrectomy

Haemorrhage into the vitreous humour may cause loss of acuity or of visual field, often of sudden onset. Alternatively changes may be more gradual due to secondary clouding and thickening of the usually transparent gel. Later scarring causes contracture with traction on the adjacent retina. Blood or other opaque tissue may be amenable to excision by vitrectomy, involving access to the vitreous via an incision in the sclera under local anaesthetic. The evacuated vitreous may be replaced with normal saline to maintain volume.

Other treatments

Intravitreous triamcinolone injection is sometimes offered to reduce leakage from diseased blood vessels particularly when the macula is affected, but the procedure needs to be repeated recurrently as its benefits are not permanent.

Other eye problems in diabetes

Rubeotic glaucoma

Rubeosis is another name for the proliferation of blood vessels in response to growth factors triggered by hypoxia. When this occurs in the vessels of the anterior chamber, neovascularisation may disrupt the outflow of aqueous humour at the angle, causing a rise in intra-ocular pressure. This can lead over time to a secondary glaucoma, with damage to visual fields and acuity. The screening programme for diabetic retinopathy in the UK does not include a measurement of intra-ocular pressure. However, people with diabetes are entitled to a free eye examination annually with a commercial optician, and pressure measurement should be offered during these assessments. Patients with evidence of neovascularisation picked up during the screening programme will be referred on for further ophthalmological assessment, and pressure measurement will be provided in this setting. In addition to

Macular Thickness:Macular cube 512 x 128

OD ◯ | ⬤ OS

Figure 13.9 Ocular Coherence Tomography (OCT) has improved the assessment of diabetic retinopathy, and here demonstrates macular oedema. (Images courtesy of Mr Gary Misson, Warwick Hospital.)

glaucoma that is secondary to rubeosis, people with diabetes are more prone to primary chronic (open angle) glaucoma than the general population.

Retinal detachment

This is a result of accumulation of fluid between the neural and pigmented retinal layers. As discussed above, fibrosis of the vitreous humour next to the retina promotes this process particularly in those with established proliferative retinopathy. A peripheral detachment may produce a field defect of gradual or sudden onset. This may or may not be noticed by the patient, but is typically heralded by a sensation of bright flashing lights. Traction with or without actual detachment may affect the macula (as discussed above) to produce acute deterioration in acuity.

Cataract

Cataract is common in diabetes, and is worsened by poor glycaemic control. The treatment is the same as for the general population.

Retinal vein occlusion

The retinal vein may become occluded, particularly if hyperglycaemia is sufficient to produce hyperviscosity. Occlusion of the central retinal vein causes catastrophic unilateral loss of vision, or more commonly a branch retinal occlusion causes loss of visual field. Associated haemorrhage, oedema and closure of the capillary circulation are typical, and complicate the picture. Fluoroscein angiography may help to determine whether spontaneous resolution is likely or whether focal laser treatment to seal off leaking vessels is required.

Figure 13.10 Scarring resulting from laser therapy in the peripheral retina (photograph courtsey of Dr Sailesh Sankar, consultant Physician, University Hospital, Coventry).

Diabetic optic neuropathy

This is a rare complication of diabetes, causing swelling and loss of function of the optic nerve, with progressive loss of acuity.

Ocular muscle palsies

People with diabetes may develop an ocular muscle palsy as an acute or subacute neuropathic event. This classically affects the third cranial (oculomotor) nerve, producing an outward and downward gaze due to weakness of adduction and unopposed action of the superior oblique. There may be an associated ptosis. In diabetes where the cause is ischaemic the pupillary reflex may be spared.

Living with diabetic retinopathy

Patients whose acuity or visual field is permanently affected require a lot of support. The first issue concerns driving ability and other safety issues. The Driving and Vehicle Licensing Authority (DVLA) issue regularly updated guidance on the medical standards of fitness to drive. For those more seriously affected, low vision clinics are available to help manage everyday self-care and promote independence. Loss of role in the home, work place and in society at large is potentially devastating and requires a proactive approach to individual support to minimise the impact on quality of life.

Summary

Modern ophthalmological techniques including laser therapy represent a major victory in the ongoing battle against diabetes. Combined with effective retinopathy screening programmes they are progressively reducing risk of visual loss. Liaison between primary and secondary care, clearly defined referral pathways, and patient education are vital if the benefits of these techniques are to be maximised. The assessment of visual symptoms in diabetes is complex and patients must have ready access to specialist expertise for the assessment of any unexpected change in acuity. The infrastructure required to provide high-quality care is largely only available in industrialised countries, meanwhile diabetes prevalence is escalating elsewhere. Responding to this escalation and its impact on the visual health of the global community is a major challenge for the coming decades.

Further reading

Diabetic Retinopathy Study Group. Photocoagulation treatment of proliferative diabetic retinopathy: the second report of diabetic retinopathy study findings. *Ophthalmology* 1978;**85**:82–106.

DVLA. 'At a glance' Guide to medical standards of fitness to drive. Available at: http://www.dvla.gov.uk/medical/ataglance.aspx

Early Treatment of Diabetic Retinopathy Study Group. Photocoagulation for diabetic macular edema. Early Treatment Diabetic Retinopathy Study. *Arch Ophthalmol* 1985;**103**:1796–806.

Retinopathy Vitrectomy Study Report 2. *Arch Ophthalmol* 1985;**103**:1644–52.

Royal College of Ophthalmologists. Guidelines for Diabetic Retinopathy. 2005. Available at: http://www.rcophth.ac.uk/docs/publications/published-guidelines/DiabeticRetinopathyGuidelines2005.pdf

The Diabetic Retinopathy Vitrectomy Study Research Group. Early vitrectomy for severe vitreous hemorrhage in diabetic retinopathy. Two-year results of a randomized trial. *Arch Ophthalmol* 1985;**103**(11):1644–52.

The Wisconsin Epidemiologic Study of Diabetic Retinopathy. XIV. Ten-year incidence and progression of diabetic retinopathy. *Arch Ophthalmol* 1994; **112**:1217–28.

The Diabetic Foot

Tim Holt[1] and Sudhesh Kumar[2]

[1]Health Sciences Research Institute, Warwick Medical School, University of Warwick, Coventry, UK
[2]Clinical Sciences Research Institute, Warwick Medical School, University of Warwick; and WISDEM, University Hospital, Coventry, UK

OVERVIEW

- Foot complications of diabetes are common and include arterial insufficiency and peripheral neuropathy, which can readily lead to ulceration

- Foot ulcers may be associated with deep infection and put the patient at risk of osteomyelitis and systemic sepsis

- Maintaining foot health demands a proactive approach involving regular checks and patient education, which should be part of routine surveillance

- Development of an 'at risk' foot justifies more frequent assessment

- Conservative measures include removal of callus, desloughing, pressure relief casts, surgical debridement, abscess drainage, and revascularisation

- Local care pathways for managing foot complications should be well understood to ensure prompt action and reduce the need for amputation

Introduction

Foot complications are a serious threat to patients with diabetes (Figure 14.1) and must always be treated energetically. Three major factors are vascular disease, peripheral neuropathy and raised risk of infection. These may threaten not only the limb in question but also the life of the individual, and regular surveillance and early intervention (particularly when infection intervenes) are essential. Around 50% of non-traumatic foot amputations are carried out on people with diabetes. Foot problems are perhaps the most preventable complication of diabetes, but require coordinated teamwork, including education of the patient and carers.

The three risk factors

Vascular insufficiency

Peripheral vascular disease is often asymptomatic until a well-established stage. Ischaemia reduces the immunological response to infection, delays healing and raises the likelihood of anaerobic infection in the deeper tissues.

Neuropathy

Peripheral neuropathy reduces light touch sensation putting the foot at risk of unnoticed trauma, and also impairs proprioception, leading to deformity and swelling of the joints. These problems can mask deeper foot sepsis, which should always be suspected when apparently superficial infection fails to heal. Neuropathy is extremely common (up to 50% of type 2 patients), but in many of these it produces no symptoms and can only be excluded through physical examination. Autonomic neuropathy is less common, but may cause reduction in sweating with dryness of the skin, promoting fissuring and ulceration.

Infection

Infection may be obvious superficially, or may be deeper, where it can invade bone, form abscesses, promote gangrene and produce systemic sepsis.

> "While mild infections are relatively easily treated, moderate infections may be limb threatening, and severe infections may be life threatening"
> International Diabetes Federation Consensus Guidelines on the Management and Prevention of the Diabetic Foot, 2003

Figure 14.1 Necrotic ulcer on the second toe with proximal erythema and swelling (photograph courtesy of Mr G Deogan, University Hospital, Coventry).

ABC of Diabetes, 6th edition. By T. Holt and S. Kumar.
Published 2010 by Blackwell Publishing.

Patterns of presentation

Whilst the factors often co-exist, two major patterns are seen (all photographs courtsey of Mr G Deogan, University Hospital, Coventry).

The neuropathic foot

Where neuropathy predominates the problems tend to occur at the pressure areas on the plantar surfaces, and ulcers are usually preceded by callus formation on the sole. Neuropathic feet (Figures 14.2 and 14.3) are typically warm with easily palpable pulses due to reduction of sympathetic tone on the arteries, but reduced sensation is present on microfilament testing. Distortion and swelling of the joints (Charcot's joints) may be present. Occasionally, severe neuropathy may cause oedema of the feet and lower legs.

The ischaemic or neuro-ischaemic foot

Where arterial insufficiency is the major factor the foot is often cool to touch and pulses are reduced or absent. Hair growth

Figure 14.4 Gangrenous ulceration in a neuro-ischaemic foot.

may be reduced although this sign is rather non-specific in older patients. If ischaemia becomes critical, the foot is typically pink and painful and urgent action is then required. Ischaemic ulcers are usually distal and on the margins of the feet rather than the soles (Figure 14.4). They are not necessarily related to callosities, in contrast to purely neuropathic ulcers. But frequently, neuropathy and ischaemia co-exist (the 'neuro-ischaemic foot', Figure 14.4), complicating assessment and this overlap should always be borne in mind.

Regular surveillance

All patients with diabetes should have a thorough foot examination at least annually, and in those with signs of complications or 'at-risk' features this frequency should be increased. The examination should include, as a minimum, the following:

- **Inspection of the general health of the feet.** Signs of deformity, hair loss, loss of skin integrity, loss of sweating, swelling of joints, callosities, nail health, fungal infection between the toes and in the nails. Deformity or swelling may suggest an underlying Charcot's joint (see Figure 14.6). Callosities suggest abnormal distribution of weight over the sole, which may indicate peripheral neuropathy
- **Assessment of vascular sufficiency.** Temperature of the skin, detection of dorsalis pedis and posterior tibial pulses, capillary return at the toes
- **Assessment of neurological integrity.** Light touch sensation using a 10 g nylon microfilament device at all of the 'at risk' areas (see Figure 14.5) and vibration sense at the great toe and ankle. Achilles tendon reflex

Problems identified during a surveillance examination should be actioned accordingly (Boxes 14.1 and 14.2). Ulceration, however small, requires immediate active management. It is estimated that 4–10% of the population with diabetes has a foot ulcer. Eighty-five per cent of foot amputations in people with diabetes occur following the development of an ulcer.

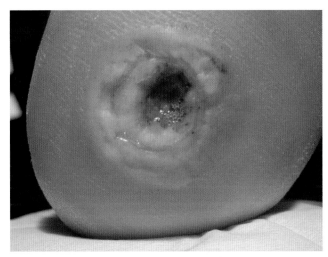

Figure 14.2 Deep heel ulceration in a neuropathic foot.

Figure 14.3 Pressure from tight footwear on insensitive toes has caused calluses now ulcerating superficially.

(a)

(b)

Figure 14.5 Patient having foot examined with 10 g microfilament (photographs courtesy of Mr G Deogan, University Hospital, Coventry).

Box 14.1 **Doppler assessment**

A suspicion of arterial insufficiency may be followed up by Doppler assessment to measure the Ankle Brachial Pressure Index (ABPI). This is a measure of the ratio of systolic pressures at the posterior tibial and brachial pulses. It should be carried out by professionals trained in the technique, and both inter- and intra-observer variability is a problem. Values greater than 1.0 are either normal or may suggest calcified vessels in the leg, particularly if greater than 1.2 (due to medial sclerosis raising the systolic pressure at the ankle). Values <0.9 suggest ischaemia and <6.0 severe ischaemia

Box 14.2 **How urgent is the foot problem?**

Referral pathways should be organised with appropriate priority:

Callus on soles
Anaesthetic areas with no
  ulceration
Fungal infection
	Routine referral to specialist
	  podiatrist

Callus with evidence of haemorrhage	Urgent referral to podiatrist
Ulceration without infection	Referral to foot clinic within 48 hours

Ulceration with infection	Same day appointment at foot clinic,
	  or admission if there are signs of
	  systemic sepsis

Ischaemia	

An absent foot pulse picked up at routine surveillance with no symptoms or associated foot problems should if considered significant, be followed up with reassessment every 3 months. Symptoms of vascular insufficiency (intermittent claudication, non-acutely cold foot) should trigger a 'soon' referral to a vascular surgeon. Rest pain requires an urgent same day referral, and an acutely cold, painful, pulseless foot requires immediate transfer to hospital by ambulance 'nil by mouth'

If there are no acute problems requiring immediate action then each foot should be classified according to its risk level, using the

Table 14.1 IDF risk categorisation system for organising review intervals.

IDF Risk categorisation system

Category	Risk profile	Check-up frequency
0	No sensory neuropathy	Once a year
1	Sensory neuropathy	Once every 6 months

2	Sensory neuropathy and signs of
	  peripheral vascular disease and/or
	  foot deformities
		Once every 3 months

3	Previous ulcer	Once every 1–3 months

IDF risk categorisation system (Table 14.1 and Box 14.3). This can be used to determine the appropriate frequency of further examinations. Patient education should be offered at every routine check (Boxes 14.4, 14.5 and 14.6).

Box 14.3 **IDF risk factors**

Previous ulcer/amputation
Lack of social contact
Lack of education
Impaired protective sensation (monofilaments)
Impaired vibration perception
Absent Achilles tendon reflex
Callus
Foot deformities
Inappropriate footwear

Box 14.4 **International Diabetes Federation: Five cornerstones of the management of the diabetic foot**

Regular inspection and examination of the foot at risk
Identification of the foot at risk
Education of patient, family and healthcare providers
Appropriate footwear
Treatment of non-ulcerative pathology

From *Diabetes/Metabolism Research and Reviews* 2008;**24**(Suppl. 1):S181–7

Charcot's joint

Loss of proprioceptive function leads to abnormal weight distribution in the ankle joint or the small joints of the foot. Initially this produces wearing and degeneration at the articular surfaces, but later the joint may become distorted and dysfunctional. The final stage of this process is a 'Charcot's joint', which is swollen and disfigured externally and disorganised internally. Reduced awareness of trauma together with disordered movements put the patient at high risk of pressure ulceration particularly if footwear is not adequate. The internal arch of the foot falls and ulceration at this site is common (Figure 14.6).

Treatment of diabetic foot complications

Importance of early referral

Once a problem is identified the patient must access the necessary expertise for energetic treatment and follow-up. This will usually involve a specialist foot clinic and all primary care clinicians must be clear regarding referral pathways. The foot clinic may be community-based but should have close links with surgical facilities.

Figure 14.6 Classic Charcot's mid-foot ulcer following collapse of the foot arches.

A major cause of ulcers failing to heal is delay in starting appropriate treatment including debridement, by which time infection that might have been treated conservatively has penetrated the deeper tissues, causing necrosis and threatening the viability of the limb. Treatment options listed include both conservative and surgical approaches (Box 14.7).

Is the ulcer infected and if so, how severely?

The first decision is over whether or not a foot ulcer or wound is infected (Figure 14.7). Next, the depth and severity of infection must be assessed (Box 14.8). These answers will determine the need for antibiotics, the choice of antibiotic, the route of administration and setting in which they are given, and the need and timing of surgical

Figure 14.7 Neglected paronychia of the right great toenail with invasive infection and ulceration of proximal tissue.

Figure 14.8 Extensive spreading cellulitis from a distal area of superficial ulceration.

intervention if appropriate. In addition to clinical examination, x-rays to exclude underlying osteomyelitis and blood tests looking for leukocytosis or other inflammatory markers may be required. However, patients with diabetes may not produce the usual response to infection and the absence of raised inflammatory markers does not exclude infection.

Box 14.8 **Signs of foot wound infection in diabetes**

Local:	Systemic:	Radiographic:
Pain	Fever	Osteomyelitis on x-ray
Tenderness	Rigors	
Eythema	Confusion	
Cellulitis	Hyperglycaemia	
Odour	Leukocytosis	
Necrosis	Raised inflammatory markers, e.g. C-reactive protein	
Gangrene		

Deep infection in the foot spaces must always be suspected whenever the patient does not respond to apparently appropriate therapy, when there are signs of systemic illness, or when signs of inflammation are present at some distance from the wound or ulcer

Antibiotic therapy

Gram-positive organisms including staphylococci and streptococci are usually responsible for superficial foot infections, whilst deeper infection may be associated with more than one pathogen, including anaerobic and Gram-negative organisms (Figure 14.8). Treatment of deep foot infection will usually require surgical removal of infected tissue, and antibiotics alone are unlikely to be adequate. Identification of the responsible pathogen is important but will take time and this should not delay the commencement of antibiotic treatment. Ideally, the infected tissue itself should be cultured following debridement but by this time the patient will usually have started empirical therapy and swabs including actual pus if present

(rather than ulcer slough) should be sent for microbiological analysis at the first opportunity. Antibiotic therapy is adjusted according to culture results and may need to be continued until the ulcer has healed (Table 14.2 and Box 14.9).

Table 14.2 International Diabetes Federation: Suggested systemic antibiotic regimens for treating diabetic foot infections.

Severity of infection	Usual pathogen(s)	Potential regimens
Non-severe (oral for entire course)		
No complicating features	GPC	S-S pen; 1 G Ceph
Recent antibiotic therapy	GPC ± GNR	FQ, β-L-ase
Drug allergies		Clindamycin; FQ; T/S
Severe (intravenous until stable, then switch to oral equivalent)		
No complicating features	GPC2 ± GNR	β-L-ase; 2/3 G Ceph
Recent antibiotic/ necrosis	GPC + GNR/ anaerobes	3/4 G Ceph; FQ + Clindamycin
Life-threatening (prolonged intravenous)		
MRSA unlikely	GPC + GNR + anaerobes	Carbapenem; Clindamycin Aminoglycoside
MRSA likely		Glycopeptide or linezolid + 3/4 G Ceph or FQ + metronidazole

Given at usual recommended doses for serious infections; modify for azotemia, etc., based on theoretical considerations and available clinical trials. A high local prevalence of methicillin resistance among staphylococci may require using vancomycin or other appropriate anti-staphylococcal agents active against these organisms.
1 G Ceph, first generation cephalosporins (e.g. cephalexin, cefazolin); 2/3/4 G Ceph, 2nd/3rd/4th generation cephalosporins (e.g. cefoxitin, ceftazidime, cefepime); β-L-ase, lactam- β lactamase-β inhibitor (e.g. amoxicillin/clavulanate, piperacillin/tazobactam); FQ, fluoroquinolones (e.g. ciprofloxacin, levofloxacin); GNR, gram-negative rod; GPC, gram-positive cocci; S-S pen, semi-synthetic (anti-staphylococcal) penicillin (e.g. flucloxacillin, oxacillin); T/S, trimethoprim/sulfamethoxazole. Carbapenem, e.g. imipenem/cilastatin, meropenem, ertapenem; aminoglycoside, e.g. gentamicin, tobramycin, amikacin; glycopeptides, e.g. vancomycin, teicoplanin.
Reproduced with permission from the IDF International Consensus of the Diabetic Foot, the Practical Guidelines (1999) and Supplements (2003).

Conservative management

Removal of callus

The finding of callus should lead to a referral to a chiropodist experienced in treating the feet of people with diabetes. In the absence of ulceration this can be done less urgently but the availability of this service is an essential component of the team management of diabetes.

Under the UK's National Health Service, podiatry and chiropody for diabetic feet (and other medical conditions) has become prioritised at the expense of general foot care in the older population without diabetes. This reflects the importance of professional treatment of early foot complications, including callus formation, which should never be 'self-managed'

Desloughing of ulcers using maggots

Removal of the slough and debris at the base of a diabetic foot ulcer may be achieved using maggots (Figure 14.9). This may be more effective than other means of desloughing and leaves the ulcer in a clean state ready to start healing.

Pressure relief casts

Ulcers often occur at the site of pressure, on the balls of the feet, the heel, or elsewhere on the sole. They are unlikely to heel if they continue to be exposed to this pressure. Scotchcast dressings with a hole over the ulcer are fitted to ensure that pressure is relieved in this area. It is essential that such casts are properly fitted to avoid new ulcers forming elsewhere on the foot. Bedrest may also be necessary to assist healing, but immobility carries its own risk.

Surgical intervention

Debridement and abscess drainage

Surgical debridement is often required to remove necrotic tissue. This in a sense is a 'conservative' measure in that it helps to reduce/prevent the need for amputation. Necrotic tissue acts like a foreign body, delaying healing, harbouring infection and making extension of infection, osteomyelitis and systemic sepsis more likely. In addition to debridement, other surgical measures include drainage of foot abscesses (which may require access to the deep foot spaces) (Figure 14.10).

Osteomyelitis underlying infected, ulcerated skin is a common complication and should be actively excluded through plain radiography (Figure 14.11) in all cases of deep or resistant infection. It often requires surgical excision and its presence will influence the choice, route of administration and duration of antibiotic therapy.

Revascularisation and limb salvage

Revascularisation should preferably occur prior to the development of an ulcer in a patient with peripheral vascular disease (Figure 14.12), but often ulceration is the first symptom of a silent background process. Where ulceration is established, angioplasty, bypass or reconstruction to the major vessels may greatly improve the chances of healing. Revascularisation is required urgently in the case of the critically ischaemic foot, requiring inpatient management.

Amputation

Amputation is indicated when conservative management fails, when persistent deep infection threatens systemic sepsis or progressive gangrene (Figure 14.13), or when rest pain is poorly controlled.

Figure 14.9 Maggot therapy.

Figure 14.10 Probing a deep sinus beneath a neuropathic ulcer.

Figure 14.11 Radiograph of osteomyelitis.

Figure 14.13 Extensive ulceration with infection and gangrene preceded this patient's below knee amputation.

Figure 14.14 Clean wound following amputation of the left little toe. Note the callosities and neuropathic ulceration on the sole.

When this is necessary, the limb must be assessed to determine the viability of proximal tissue. Adequate vascular supply is essential for healing, and if amputation is not extensive enough this healing may fail. Toe amputation is usually unsuccessful when there is significant ischaemia present, but may be an option in the purely neuropathic foot, or when revascularisation is successful (Figure 14.14). If so, conservation of the great toe may reduce the impact on limb function post-operatively. A dry, necrotic toe (Figure 14.15) may be left to 'auto-amputate' if infection is not an issue.

Figure 14.12 Radiograph of atheromatous narrowing.

Figure 14.15 Dry necrosis of the distal right great toe.

Figure 14.16 Successful healing following amputation of the third and fourth toes.

Rehabilitation

The patient must also be assessed in a more holistic way to determine the options for rehabilitation. Some younger, fitter patients may manage with a prosthetic limb and regain walking mobility following limb amputation (Figure 14.16). Older, frailer or obese patients may not have this option, and are more likely to become wheelchair-dependent. These social consequences should be discussed with the patient and family if there is time before the decisions are made, even if amputation is inevitable. The psychological response to amputation is complex. For some, it has been compared to a bereavement. Involvement of the patient and carers in management decisions helps in this adjustment. Apart from the human costs of amputation and resulting disability, the health economic effects justify an intensive, proactive approach to ulcer management and follow-up, even in countries with less developed resources.

Prognosis

Amputation often signifies the end stage of advanced complications, and amputees not only have a high risk of future amputation in the other limb but also a high all-cause mortality rate in the year following the operation.

Further reading

International Diabetes Federation. *International consensus on the diabetic foot*, 2003.

Jeffcoate W, Lipsky BA, Berendt AR, *et al.* on behalf of the three systematic review working parties of the International Working Group on the Diabetic Foot. Unresolved issues in the management of ulcers of the foot in diabetes. *Diabetic Med* 2008;**25**:1380–9.

CHAPTER 15

Diabetic Neuropathy

Tim Holt[1] and Sudhesh Kumar[2]

[1]Health Sciences Research Institute, Warwick Medical School, University of Warwick, Coventry, UK
[2]Clinical Sciences Research Institute, Warwick Medical School, University of Warwick; and WISDEM, University Hospital, Coventry, UK

OVERVIEW

- Diabetic neuropathy is a very common complication of diabetes

- Peripheral neuropathy is often painful and this is a disabling complication, increasing the risk of foot ulceration due to impaired sensation

- Good control of hyperglycaemia, blood pressure and dyslipidaemia is important for prevention and reducing progression of neuropathy

- Autonomic neuropathy causes a number of problems including gastroparesis, gustatory sweating, postural hypotension and diarrhoea

- Neuropathy may combine with vascular insufficiency to produce erectile dysfunction

- Erectile dysfunction usually responds to drug therapy and other treatments

---

Introduction

There are many forms of diabetic neuropathy but the commonest form is a peripheral sensorimotor neuropathy that affects the feet first. Poorly controlled hyperglycaemia, uncontrolled hypertension and dyslipidaemia are associated with the development and progression of neuropathy. Excess alcohol consumption can also be a contributory factor. Chronic peripheral neuropathy due to diabetes is a progressive condition and can be expected to worsen over time. This is in contrast to acute neuropathies and especially cranial mononeuropathies that tend to recover. Mononeuropathies result from microvascular disease. Compression neuropathies are also common in diabetes and the commonest form of such neuropathy is carpal tunnel syndrome, although foot drop and ulnar neuropathy are also occasionally seen in patients with diabetes.

Peripheral neuropathy

Presentation

The commonest symptom is pain or altered sensation in the feet. Allodynia is common and symptoms include a sensation of feet feeling cold or a feeling of pins and needles in the feet. Patients

---

ABC of Diabetes, 6th edition. By T. Holt and S. Kumar.
Published 2010 by Blackwell Publishing.

may complain that their bedclothes irritate the feet and these symptoms may keep the patient up at night. In contrast some patients experience a feeling of complete numbness. In both these cases, reduced sensation in the feet is a hazard to the patient who is then at risk of injury, ulceration and ensuing infection.

Neuropathy can affect both type 1 and type 2 patients. In patients with type 1 diabetes it is seen after many years of diabetes. In type 2 patients it may be present at the time of diagnosis itself. Patients on high doses of metformin may occasionally present with a neuropathy due to Vitamin B12 deficiency, therefore, if in doubt, check serum Vitamin B12.

During the early stages, clinical examination may not reveal any significant abnormality. Once clinically significant neuropathy is present, it is revealed by impairment of pressure perception tested with a 10 g monofilament, reduced vibration perception tested using a 128 Hz tuning fork and absent ankle reflexes. Nerve conduction studies may reveal abnormalities in a significant proportion of patients with diabetes, who often do not have any symptoms and are not at high risk of foot ulceration. This test is more useful when compression neuropathy is suspected.

Tight control of glycaemia with insulin may reduce the progression of neuropathy. Several drugs have been developed and tested in trials, but none have so far been shown to alter the progression of neuropathy other than control of diabetes and related risk factors.

Patients with peripheral neuropathy may also experience reduced sweating in the feet, which is a feature of autonomic dysfunction. The dryness of skin that results may predispose to foot ulceration. Regular application of intensive care Vaseline or other skin emollients help to keep the skin healthy.

Treatment

Tight control of the principal risk factors, hyperglycaemia, blood pressure and lipids may help reduce progression. There is no specific therapy that has proven to be effective in altering the natural history of neuropathy, thus far. Painful neuropathy can be extremely difficult to live with and the clinician should be sympathetic to the plight of the patient, and offer symptomatic treatment (Box 15.1). When it fails to respond to simple analgesics like paracetamol, tricyclic antidepressants, the newer antidepressant duloxetine or anti-epileptic agents such as gabapentin or carbamazepine may be helpful. Opiates may sometimes be required for pain that does not respond to other measures.

Box 15.1 **Treatment options for painful neuropathy**

Topical agents:

Topical capsaicin cream
Opsite dressing to reduce contact pain
Lignocaine-impregnated patches (Versatis)

Oral agents:

Simple analgesia – e.g. paracetamol
Amitriptyline (10–25 mg at night, increased if needed up to 75 mg)
Duloxetine 60–120 mg daily
Pregabalin (150 mg/day in two to three divided doses, increased if needed after 3–7 days to 300 mg/day in two to three divided doses, then further increased if needed after 7 days to maximum 600 mg/day in two to three divided doses)
Gabapentin (300 mg on day one, then 300 mg twice a day on day two, then 300 mg three times a day on day three, increased according to response in steps of 300 mg/day to maximum 1.8 g daily)
Carbamazepine, sodium valproate, topiramate
Opiates if pain intractable (but high risk of dependency)

Acute painful neuropathies

These tend to present acutely and recover over the course of 6–18 months. These are more commonly seen in patients with type 2 diabetes and are thought to be due to vascular disease. Effective pain relief is required, as is good control of glycaemia and associated risk factors. Application of Opsite may help to relieve pain in these cases.

Autonomic neuropathy

Autonomic neuropathy occurs as a long-term complication of diabetes and is associated with long duration of diabetes and a history of poor glycaemic control.

Postural hypotension

Even in those with a clinically detectable drop in blood pressure of more than 20 mmHg, symptoms are unusual. A drop in blood pressure of more than 30 mmHg is often seen in those patients who complain of dizziness while standing. The patient's blood pressure should be checked at least 2 minutes after standing from a supine position. Unexplained hypoglycaemia and new onset of postural hypotension may also be due to Addison's disease in patients with type 1 diabetes. When suspected, this diagnosis should be excluded by a short synacthen test.

For patients with symptoms, the treatment should start with exclusion of drugs that can aggravate the problem. Where there are significant symptoms, it may be necessary to ask the patient to increase salt intake. Fludrocortisone may be prescribed for symptomatic postural hypotension after the above measures have been tried.

Gustatory sweating

Profuse facial sweating, especially after eating something savoury is a symptom of autonomic neuropathy. Often an explanation is all

that is needed, but if treatment is required, glypyrrolate cream can be prepared for the patient by any hospital pharmacy department. The cream is then applied to the affected areas.

Autonomic diarrhoea

Nocturnal diarrhoea in patients with long-standing diabetes may be due to autonomic neuropathy. Here exclusion of other bowel problems, especially conditions such as coeliac or pancreatic disease is important. Autonomic neuropathy can be established by testing for cardiovascular autonomic dysfunction (Figure 15.1). Treatment can be given in the form of codeine phosphate, but doxycycline 50 mg given daily for 3–4 days and thereafter once every other day for 2 weeks is often effective in many patients.

Diabetic gastroparesis

Gastroparesis leading to vomiting is rare, although milder forms are not uncommon. Patients may report vomiting contents of meals consumed more than 24 hours earlier. Presence of a gastric splash on examination is another clue to the diagnosis. The patient should then be referred for investigation and radiolabelled porridge studies can help establish the diagnosis.

Pro-kinetic anti-emetics are often used including metoclopramide. In severe cases where the patient suffers intractable vomiting, percutaneous endoscopic jejunostomy may be required.

Other autonomic neuropathic problems

Severe constipation requiring colectomy is now exceptionally rare but still seen from time to time. Other complications due to autonomic neuropathy may include neurogenic bladder resulting in urinary retention. This may eventually require treatment by self-catheterisation, two to three times daily. Erectile dysfunction and retrograde ejaculation are also problems related to autonomic

Figure 15.1 Heart rate changes in a normal subject (left) and a patient with autonomic neuropathy (right) showing loss of heart rate variation in autonomic neuropathy during deep breathing, at six breaths a minute (top), and loss of "overshoot" cardiac acceleration on standing (bottom).

neuropathy. Respiratory arrests may also occur. This is important when patients undergo surgery with anaesthesia.

Erectile dysfunction

Erectile dysfunction is common in men over the age of 50 years. In men with diabetes, it is more common and occurs at a younger age, causing considerable distress to both the patient and his partner. Neuropathy, vascular disease, alcohol and drugs are the main underlying organic causes for erectile dysfunction in patients with diabetes. However, as in those without diabetes, in many it has an underlying psychogenic basis. The anxiety that this loss of function is due to diabetes makes the problem worse.

Clinical assessment

Patients complaining of erectile dysfunction should undergo a full clinical examination including examination of the external genitalia. Gradual onset of erectile dysfunction with loss of nocturnal erections in someone with long-standing diabetes is likely to be due to diabetes. On the other hand sudden onset and intermittent symptoms and the preservation of nocturnal erections suggest an underlying psychological basis instead. In these cases, exploring any difficulties in the patients' relationships or any major work or financial stress may reveal the underlying reason. The presence of neuropathy, peripheral and/or autonomic makes neurogenic impotence more likely. The presence of significant vascular disease suggests that there may be vascular insufficiency. Many drugs taken with diabetes can cause erectile dysfunction and excess alcohol intake is often a significant contributor to the problem. Symptoms and signs of hypogonadism should also be looked for.

Investigation

Thyroid function tests and free testosterone should be checked. Serum prolactin should be measured if free testosterone is low. These tests are usually normal in patients with diabetes and erectile dysfunction. In patients with normal serum testosterone there is no value in prescribing testosterone supplements although patients may often request this.

Management of erectile dysfunction

First, it is important to explain the cause to the patient and his partner and also provide reassurance that it can usually be effectively treated. This is especially important if no obvious underlying cause is found and psychological factors are thought to be likely to have caused the symptom. Patients with major psychological problems that have been identified during the consultation or with significant relationship problems may benefit from being referred to a psychologist or relationship counsellor.

Phosphodiesterase inhibitors

First line drug treatment includes oral therapies such as phosphodiesterase inhibitors. Many men can be successfully treated with

oral therapy such as Sildenafil, Vardenafil or Tadalafil. The patient is asked to take the tablet between 30 minutes to 1 hour before sexual activity if using Sildenafil, whilst some preparations can be taken up to 24 hours earlier (Tadalafil). These treatments are contra-indicated in those taking nitrates, those with blood pressure <90/50 mmHg, or after a recent stroke or myocardial infarction. The success of Sildenafil and other oral agents has revolutionised the treatment of erectile dysfunction and improved the lives of millions with diabetes.

Sublingual apomorphine

This is rapidly absorbed after sublingual administration and acts as a dopamine agonist. It is effective within 10–20 minutes and requires sexual stimulation to be effective. The dose ranges between 2 and 3 mg and it is effective in approximately 50% of diabetic patients suffering from erectile dysfunction.

Prostaglandin preparations
Transurethral alprostadil (MUSE)

This is applied into the urethra with an applicator provided. This modality of treatment can produce an erection after sexual stimulation.

Intracavernosal injection: alprostadil

This is less widely used since the oral therapies have become available. However, it is used as second line therapy after oral therapies have proved ineffective. Many diabetes centres and hospital neurology departments offer a service where patients are taught how to give themselves an injection avoiding the penile artery and the urethra. Bruising and priapism may complicate this therapy.

Vacuum devices

These devices have become less widely used with availability of other therapies. However, it is an option where pharmacological therapies have failed, or when venous leak is a problem. Several companies now produce vacuum devices and the patient is usually required to purchase the device. The external cylinder is fitted over the penis, a vacuum is created inside the cylinder resulting in penile engorgement, at this point an elastic ring is applied to the base of the penis that sustains the erection. This form of therapy is more often used in older patients.

Penile prostheses

Various prostheses are available that are surgically inserted into the shaft of the penis. Some sophisticated devices allow erections to be controlled by the patients, this is sometimes used in younger patients with erectile dysfunction due to organic causes.

Further reading
Tracy JA, Dyck PJ. The spectrum of diabetic neuropathies. *Phys Med Rehabil Clin N Am* 2008;**19**:1–26, v.

Unger J, Cole BE. Recognition and management of diabetic neuropathy. *Prim Care* 2007;**34**:887–913, viii.

CHAPTER 16

Psychological Issues Related to Diabetes Care

Tim Holt[1] and Sudhesh Kumar[2]

[1] Health Sciences Research Institute, Warwick Medical School, University of Warwick, Coventry, UK
[2] Clinical Sciences Research Institute, Warwick Medical School, University of Warwick; and WISDEM, University Hospital, Coventry, UK

OVERVIEW

- Psychological problems are common in people with diabetes but most can be overcome with support and education

- Diabetes is commoner in those with chronic mental illness

- Problems range from those of adjustment to more serious depressive illness and maladaptive coping behaviours

- Screening for depression using validated assessment tools should be part of routine surveillance

- Psychological health is key to successful self-management

- Family cohesion and agreement about management responsibilities improves metabolic control

---

Introduction

Earlier chapters have discussed some of the psychological issues that people with diabetes may encounter, issues with which clinicians should be familiar. There may be positive aspects such as self-efficacy, autonomy and empowerment. But there may also be more negative aspects such as the 'learned helplessness' that was mentioned in Chapter 10. Here, we discuss these in more detail including more serious disorders of psychological adjustment. We will first of all cover some of the less serious issues that most patients may encounter to some degree, before considering the serious problems that affect a small minority.

Adjusting behaviourally to the diagnosis

Diabetes may happen to anyone, and occurs no less commonly in those with pre-existing psychological or psychiatric disorders, some of which may predispose to diabetes. In type 1 patients, usually presenting in childhood, the personality is still in the developmental stage when the need for dietary discipline, frequent self-injection and blood glucose monitoring arise, all potentially disrupting this formative process (Figure 16.1). It is, therefore, not surprising that adjustment behaviours may become maladaptive, and sometimes frankly self-destructive. There is some evidence that children with diabetes are more likely to have difficulties with

information processing and learning problems, particularly those with very early diagnosis or history of severe hypoglycaemia. Poor metabolic control is associated with greater risk of a psychological diagnosis, and frequent hospital admissions lead to recurrent school absence, further disrupting education.

However, there is no one 'personality type' typical of type 1 diabetes, and most adjust remarkably well to these potential stresses, given sufficient family and peer support, as well as that of their health professionals. In fact, empowered type 1 individuals benefit from the fact that their behaviour is still flexible enough to adapt to the new requirements. This is something that older, type 2 patients typically find difficult, and in their cases it is behavioural inertia and inflexibility that are the obstacle to successful management.

Multidisciplinary behavioural interventions involving the family have been shown to improve regimen adherence and glycaemic control in type 1 children (Box 16.1), but are usually most effective when introduced soon after the diagnosis.

Box 16.1 **Components of effective behavioural interventions in children with diabetes**

Goal setting
Self-monitoring
Positive reinforcement
Behavioural contracts
Supportive parental communications
Appropriately shared responsibility for diabetes management

Needle phobia

A reluctance to pierce the skin with a sharp foreign body is of course a perfectly natural response in childhood, and also affects quite a proportion of adults. Education over the safety of injections, the use of short 6 mm needles, and a lot of practice, overcome this in the majority of patients young and old. Type 1 individuals, who rapidly become insulin-dependent, usually solve the problem fairly quickly through repeated exposure to the trigger as there is no alternative. But in older type 2 individuals it may become an unspoken reason why insulin therapy is repeatedly deferred, adding to other sources of inertia.

Demonstrating modern insulin injection technique often overcomes needle phobia, along with supportive encouragement.

ABC of Diabetes, 6th edition. By T. Holt and S. Kumar.
Published 2010 by Blackwell Publishing.

Figure 16.1 Diabetes takes some getting used to even for robust personalities.

Familiarity with the device and the injection technique on the part of the clinician is important to foster an atmosphere of confidence building. If the clinician appears under-confident or clumsy then this will amplify any anxiety on the patient's side.

A minority of patients remain excessively anxious about insulin injections. Children may become dependent on their parents administering the insulin, a pattern that is, of course, necessary if diabetes occurs in early childhood, but in older children should be resisted to promote eventual independence.

Dishonesty in recording blood glucose results

The tendency of patients to fabricate blood glucose results to placate their clinician is now well known, and there is evidence that this behaviour occurs among widely differing patient subgroups. One celebrity patient made it his New Year's resolution to not invent quite so many self-monitored results. Some patients wish to disguise the fact that they have not taken any readings at all, or only a few. In these cases the give-away may be the use of the same pen or pencil to write all of the results down at the same time, although some may have appropriately accessed the meter's memory and written all the results out in one go for the clinician's benefit. A check on the meter's memory may confirm this, or may reveal that the reported results on the profile are a selected sample. Before confronting a patient for abusing time and trust, it is worth stepping back and in each individual's case trying to work out why it has happened from their perspective.

In the case of the person who is not self-monitoring despite advice to do so, why are they not sufficiently motivated? The missing link here may be their ability to make sense of the patterns, resulting in the 'learned helplessness' phenomenon described in Chapter 10. A discussion needs to take place over the purpose of the self-monitoring, whether it is for the clinician's or the patient's benefit, who should be responsible for analysing the results and making adjustments, and the extent to which this should be done using the retrospective rather than prospective approach (see Chapter 10). Time invested in teaching the patient some simple rules for interpreting the data and making dose adjustments, provided

they are able to learn these skills, goes much further than a simple reprimand that will further damage their feelings of self-efficacy as well as the clinician-patient relationship.

Patients may have hidden agendas that only come to light on active questioning. Driving safety, employment issues and health insurance are all plausible and understandable (if not excusable) bases for deceptive behaviour. The answer, again, is to keep 'on the same side' and avoid the 'Armande' response (Chapter 3), where even adults may occasionally develop a juvenile rebelliousness that is uncharacteristic of the rest of their behaviour.

'Food addiction'

The pre-existing psychological or psychiatric history of the individual may be very relevant to the patient's adjustment to the diabetes diagnosis, and their coping mechanisms. Type 2 diabetes occurs more often in overweight people. Many of these have simply developed bad eating habits in a culture that is increasingly sedentary and in which high calorie foods are widely available. Such people may have little or no psychological pathology, but nevertheless have a serious physical problem that must be overcome by psychological means. A few are obese because of an abnormal attitude towards food, and in some the term 'food addiction' might be appropriate.

Food addiction has been defined as 'eating types and amounts of foods that seem to contrast with a person's intentions to make moderate and 'sensible' food choices.' However, it is a matter of controversy whether this term is appropriate to people who eat excessively. Nevertheless, those in the severely obese category may benefit from psychological referral, to explore and address underlying reasons for their eating behaviour, including body image, the meaning of food in their lives, and their response to hunger and satiety.

Depression and diabetes

Whilst all patients are likely at times to feel burdened by the prognostic implications of their diagnosis, a significant proportion will develop potentially serious depressive illnesses. This problem is common enough that it should be actively sought by questioning during regular diabetes reviews, as should some of the issues that may contribute to it, such as erectile dysfunction. These problems, unlike biochemical indices, are difficult to measure but represent a large component of the person's quality of life.

Depression is a common finding in chronic disease generally, but in the case of diabetes has a particularly significant impact on the mean health score (Figure 16.2).

Depression screening has been introduced into regular diabetes surveillance in the UK through the Quality and Outcomes Framework (see Chapter 18). It uses a validated screening tool involving two questions, following any positive responses with a more detailed questionnaire to assess severity. Three such questionnaires are available. The most commonly used is the PHQ-9 (Table 16.1).

'Self-defeating' behaviour

This psychological condition can affect anyone with or without diabetes. In the case of the insulin-treated individual the situation

Table 16.1 Patient Health Questionnaire (PHQ-9).

PATIENT, HEALTH QUESTIONNAIRE (PHQ-9)

NAME: _____   DATE: _____

Over the last 2 weeks, how often have you been bothered by any of the following problems? (*use* "✓" to indicate your answer)

	Not at all	Several days	More than half the days	Nearly every day
1. Little interest or pleasure in doing things			✓	
2. Feeling down, depressed, or hopeless		✓		
3. Trouble falling or staying asleep, or sleeping too much			✓	
4. Feeling tired or having little energy				✓
5. Poor appetite or overeating		✓		
6. Feeling bad about yourself – or that you are a failure or have let yourself or your family down			✓	
7. Trouble concentrating on things, such as reading the newspaper or watching television			✓	
8. Moving or speaking so slowly that other people could having noticed. Or the opposite – being so fidgety or restless that you have been moving around a lot more than usual			✓	
9. Thoughts that you would be better off dead, or of hurting yourself in some way	✓			
add colomns:		2	10	3
TOTAL:			15	

10. If you checked off any problems, how ***difficult*** have these problems made it for you to do your work, take care of things at home, or get along with other people?	Not difficult at all _____ Somewhat difficult ✓ _____ Very difficult _____ Extremely difficult _____

is serious, as the patient has control of a potentially lethal weapon among their self-sabotaging behaviours. It is a pattern that is usually established by early adulthood and may require intensive psychological treatment with close liaison between the psychologist and the diabetes team. Behavioural treatments are available, which may involve residential behavioural retraining, but the availability of such programmes is limited.

Milder forms of self-sabotage may occur in many patients, at times of disillusionment or under stressful circumstances. For some people, awaiting a forthcoming diabetes review may be stressful. It may be necessary to take this into account when assessing recent profiles. Such people typically require support to improve their self-efficacy and autonomy.

It is important to distinguish patients displaying the more benign forms, or those whose behaviour reflects an underlying depressive illness, from those whose self-defeating behaviour is a more serious primary problem affecting other areas of their lives, as the treatment approach in each case will be quite different.

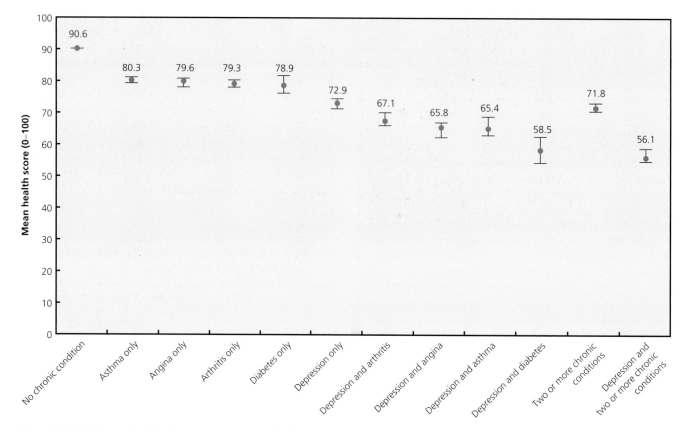

Figure 16.2 Global mean health by disease status. Reproduced with permission from Moussavi S, Chatterji S, Verdes E, *et al. Lancet* 2007;**370**:851–8.

Eating disorders in diabetes

We have mentioned above the problem of 'food addiction', in which excessive calorie intake continues way beyond energy requirements leading to severe obesity and its complications. Diabetes may often be a result rather than a cause of this abnormal behaviour.

In addition, people with established anorexia or bulimia nervosa may later develop diabetes, compounding their disordered nutritional status. These problems require co-ordinated, multidisciplinary input from physicians, diabetes nurses, psychiatrists or psychologists, and dieticians.

Therapeutic inertia

In the past, reluctance to accept insulin therapy in people with type 2 diabetes was often attributed to patient-centred issues, including their reluctance to engage in a new life pattern of daily or more frequent injections.

More recently, it has been recognised that the problem is compounded through an interaction between patient- and practitioner-centred factors. Recognising our own complicity in this process is important. We may be responsible for amplifying anxiety through our own lack of confidence with managing insulin, or simply by referring to it as if it is a desperate, last resort measure. Similarly, patients and clinicians may vacillate for months over blood pressure treatment or the addition of second or third drugs in the regimen. Patients may pick up signals from the clinician reinforcing the assumption that the need for medication simply results from failure of life-style change. Whilst life-style change is effective and should be actively promoted, such an assumption is unfair, as the majority will also need medication to achieve ideal targets (Box 16.2).

Box 16.2 **To avoid therapeutic inertia:**

- Mention the range of possible treatments early on including insulin (using positive language), preferably at one of the early appointments after the diagnosis

- Discuss the fact that whilst not needed now, insulin is often required at a later stage in type 2 diabetes, as blood glucose levels tend to become more difficult to control

- Emphasise the benefits of tight blood pressure control in diabetes, mentioning early on that two or three different drug classes are usually required to achieve this

- It will therefore not be 'their fault' if the patient eventually requires insulin and several different antihypertensive medications

- Reassure the patient that there are several different classes and many different individual antihypertensive drugs available – it is therefore likely that a suitable combination will be found for them

Figure 16.3 With support from family, friends, and health professionals many of the psychological challenges of diabetes can be overcome.

Summary

Even the most robust personalities will find diabetes a challenge, particularly type 1 patients who must adapt behaviourally over a short timescale to develop new habits and daily practices, including insulin injections. Others may feel the burden of long-term complications or a fear of them developing in the future. Many simply feel out of control, and it is through addressing this feeling that the greatest impact can be made. The empowered patient who has 'ownership' of their diabetes is likely to have improved quality of life and lower psychological morbidity (Figure 16.3). Health professionals should nurture self-efficacy in all patients whilst remaining aware of the possibility of more serious psychological problems. Depression is common in diabetes and the combination is very detrimental to quality of life. For children with diabetes, behavioural interventions should be family-centred, and preferably started soon after diagnosis where the need is evident.

Further reading

Delamater AM. Psychological care of children and adolescents with diabetes. *Pediatr Diabetes* 2007;**8**:340–8.

Lloyd CE, Dyer PH, Barnett AH. Prevalence of symptoms of depression and anxiety in a diabetes clinic population. *Diabetic Med* 2000;**17**:198–202.

Moussavi S, Chatterji S, Verdes E, *et al.* Depression, chronic disease, and decrements in health: results from the World Health Surveys. *Lancet* 2007;**370**:851–8.

Diabetes and Pregnancy

Tim Holt[1], Sudhesh Kumar[2] and Aresh Anwar[3]

[1]Health Sciences Research Institute, Warwick Medical School, University of Warwick, Coventry, UK
[2]Clinical Sciences Research Institute, Warwick Medical School, University of Warwick; and WISDEM, University Hospital, Coventry, UK
[3]University Hospital, Coventry, UK

OVERVIEW

- Pregnancy may precipitate diabetes in previously healthy but susceptible individuals

- Diabetes raises the risk of a complicated pregnancy, increasing both maternal and perinatal mortality, and the risk of congenital malformations

- Pregnancy may cause deterioration of established diabetic complications and should be avoided in those with poor glycaemic control

- Tight control of diabetes during pregnancy reduces adverse outcomes substantially

- Most patients with pre-existing diabetes will require insulin during pregnancy to achieve optimal targets if they are not already using it

- Management should be coordinated through close liaison and frequent review by the diabetes, obstetric and midwifery teams

- Follow-up of women with gestational diabetes after pregnancy is important to exclude persistent hyperglycaemia and because the lifetime risk of type 2 diabetes is high

Introduction

The standard of obstetric care for women with diabetes has seen dramatic improvements over the past few decades. Several areas however, continue to cause concern. This is reflected by morbidity and mortality in this cohort of individuals, which remains unacceptably high (Table 17.1).

Good pregnancy care starts before conception and finishes long after the birth of the baby. This form of proactive approach has been shown to help reduce the risk of complications.

Women who already have diabetes and are of childbearing age, should have pre-pregnancy counselling and optimisation of glycaemic control prior to the pregnancy. All such patients should be managed in joint diabetic pregnancy clinics where there is input from both diabetes specialist teams and obstetricians with a team of midwives. Diabetic pregnancies are considered high-risk

ABC of Diabetes, 6th edition. By T. Holt and S. Kumar.
Published 2010 by Blackwell Publishing.

pregnancies (Tables 17.1 and 17.5) and deliveries should be planned in units with appropriate neonatal care facilities.

Preconceptual management in women with pre-existing diabetes

As congenital malformations remain a major cause of morbidity, it is critical that optimal metabolic control is achieved *before* conception (Table 17.3). Unplanned pregnancies in women with diabetes should be avoided and therefore it is important to address contraception in all such women of childbearing age. This will help in planning pregnancy and optimising conditions for the best pregnancy outcome. In those mothers with evidence of diabetic complications it is important these are treated optimally prior to pregnancy. Diabetic women planning pregnancy should be helped to achieve optimal glycaemic control, preferably with HbA1c below 6.1%,

Table 17.1 Increased risks for babies of women with diabetes compared to the non-diabetic population.

Stillbirths	4.7 ×
Death of baby in first 4 weeks	2.6 ×
Major congenital anomaly	2 ×

Table 17.2 Classification of diabetes in pregnancy.

Pregnancy in patients with type 1 and type 2 diabetes	Diagnosis of diabetes predates pregnancy
Gestational diabetes	Diabetes first diagnosed in pregnancy Normally develops in second trimester (24–28 weeks) Diagnosed by oral glucose tolerance test giving a 2 hour post-challenge level ≥7.8 mmol/l

Table 17.3 Preconception checklist.

Contraception until tight control achieved (<6.1–6.5%)
Folic acid 5 mg per day
Stop teratogenic drugs – ACE inhibitors and statins in particular
Screen for complications – retinal screen, creatinine, ACR
Check thyroid function and rubella antibodies
Provide some literature – Diabetes UK website and pregnancy guide

Prepregnancy advice for diabetes

Clinics run on a regular basis at participating hospitals

- Counselling regarding benefit of prepregnancy care and importance of good glycaemic control
- Assessment of glucose control over preceding 3 months (education on importance of good control)
- Capillary blood glucose testing qds – pre breakfast and either 1 or 2 hours post meals
- Glucose targets:
  - pre meals 4–6 mmols/L (fasting 3.5–5.5 mmol/l)
  - 1 hrs post meals 4–8 mmols/L or 2 hr post meals 4–7 mmol/l
- Bloods 3 monthly:
  - U&E's
  - HbA1c (aim for HbA1c <6.5%)
- Rubella status – ensure active immunity
- Urine for Microalbuminuria
- Folic Acid 5 mgs

- Micro and Macrovascular complications discussed with referral to appropriate medical team if needed
- Medication discussed: diuretics, statins and other contraindicated medication to be stopped/changed
- Full retinal assessment with their optician and referred to ophthalmologist if needed
- Height, weight and BMI documented, dietary advice and support from Dietician
- Smoking cessation & referral if needed
- Contraception discussed and encouraged until good glucose control achieved
- Advice to contact Diabetes Specialist Nurse or Diabetes Midwife and GP after a +ve pregnancy test
- Relevant contact numbers documented for patient (eg written in glucose testing diary)

WANDA guidelines No:6. Version 2. Dated Jan 07.

Figure 17.1 Preconceptual advice for women with diabetes planning a pregnancy (provided by Dr Aresh Anwar, University Hospital, Coventry).

although this is often difficult to achieve despite intensive insulin therapy management. Women with diabetes are currently advised to take a dose of folic acid that is over ten times higher than that of women who do not have diabetes, i.e. 5 mg/day. If the above conditions are met, the congenital malformation rate is dramatically reduced to nearly that of control population levels (Figure 17.1).

Patients exposed to poor glycaemic control in the first trimester are at risk of congenital malformations although a more common scenario is for the patient with poor glycaemic control to experience recurrent miscarriages.

Those whose HbA1c is greater than 10% preconceptually should be strongly advised to avoid pregnancy. Otherwise there is a two- to fourfold increase in the congenital abnormality rate. Abnormalities include spina bifida, congenital heart disease, microcephaly and anencephaly. In women of South Asian origin in particular, consanguinity is still a major issue and this will of course increase the risk of congenital malformations by itself.

Gestational diabetes

Diabetes detected for the first time during pregnancy is known as gestational diabetes. Pregnancy is potentially 'diabetogenic' and may trigger hyperglycaemia, particularly if the patient is already at risk, for instance through family history. Babies born to women with gestational diabetes, like those with pre-existing diabetes, are larger than normal and this may affect both foetal and maternal outcomes.

These women are also therefore managed by close monitoring in a joint diabetes antenatal clinic. The WHO definition of gestational diabetes now includes those with impaired glucose tolerance during pregnancy (see Table 17.2).

Screening for gestational diabetes

Screening for gestational diabetes by glucose tolerance test is recommended in certain risk factor groups (see Box 17.1). These include obesity, family history of diabetes, older women and also women in ethnic minorities particularly South Asians, as it accounts for high rates of gestational diabetes. In those with risk factors, a glucose tolerance test is offered usually between 24 and 28 weeks of gestation. Those with a history of previous gestational diabetes should be treated as having gestational diabetes during subsequent pregnancies.

Box 17.1 **Screening for gestational diabetes**

At 28 weeks

First degree relative with diabetes (any type)
Body mass index >35 kg/m^2
Maternal age >35 years
Ethnic minority – South Asian, Afro-Caribbean, Black African
Polycystic ovary syndrome
Long-term steroids
Previous unexplained stillbirth

Previous history of macrosomia (birth weight >4.5 kg or >90th centile for gestation (on customised growth chart if available)) Polyhydramnios or foetal macrosomia in current pregnancy (>90th centile on customised growth chart)

Early screening
Previous history of gestational diabetes should have a glucose tolerance test arranged for 16–20 weeks with a repeat at 28 weeks if the first is normal

Immediate screening
Glycosuria ++ or above on two occasions (second sample within 1 week) or +++ on single occasion Urgent blood glucose if significant ketonuria

Treatment of gestational diabetes

Gestational diabetes is initially treated with diet alone and mild exercise is also encouraged. Options for treatment may include oral hypoglycaemics such as glibenclamide or metformin, but often patients require insulin. In these cases insulin or the oral hypoglycaemic agents can be stopped upon delivery.

Monitoring of the pregnant patient with diabetes

Organisation of antenatal care and frequency of reviews are summarised in Figure 17.2. HbA1c measures are important preconceptually and in the first trimester, but less useful later in pregnancy,

Diabetic Antenatal Care

Pregestational diabetes
1st Visit

- Bloods – HbA1c, U&E's, Urine for microalbuminuria
- Folic Acid 5 mgs
- Accurate Medical + Obstetric history
- Medication – STOP Statins, Diuretics, ACE Inhibiters.
- If on Oral Hypoglycaemic Agents transfer to Insulin
- Full assessment of glucose control and adjustments made
- Glucose Targets: pre-meals 4–6 mmols/L (fasting 3.5–5.5) 1hr post meal < 8mmol/l OR 2hrs post meals <7 mmols/L

- BP + Urinalysis for Protein/Ketones
- Scan arranged for 7–9 wks gestation to con. rm viability.
- Fundal screening for retinopathy
- Hypostop/ Glucagon/ instructions for treatment of hypoglycaemia
- Dietetic Advice low fat/sugar high fibre
- Smoking cessation
- Check glucose meter, check ketone testing
- Review sick day rules

Pregestational diabetes
20–34 wks

- 2 wkly visits or tailored to patient needs
- Scans – Detailed fetal and cardiac scan at 20 weeks, Fetal growth at 28 weeks.
- Bloods – 4wkly HbA1c + RBS
- Retinal screening each trimester (or opthalmologist review)
- Prompt diagnosis & treatment of: raised BP/ Pre-eclampsia/ urine and vaginal infections
- Ketoacidosis requires admission

Gestational diabetes
28–34 wks

- 2 weekly visits tailored to individual needs
- Growth scans, bloods and screening for bp/Pre-Eclampsia as above

20–34 wks

- 1–2 weekly visits
- Close monitoring of fetal movements
- Weekly assessment of fetal wellbeing liquor vol + umbilical artery Doppler scan/CTGs
- Growth scans at 34 wks then as needed
- 4 weekly HbA1c

- Prompt diagnosis & treatment of: ketoacidosis/raised BP//pre-eclampsia /urine and vaginal Infections
- Discuss delivery plan, involving Consultant Obstetrician with aim to deliver at <40 wks.
- Obstetric anaesthetic review at 34 wks
- Plan glycaemic management during and after delivery

Pregestational diabetes
Up to 20 wks

- Formal dating scan (at 11–14 weeks)
- Pregnancy booking bloods
- Review of glycaemic targets
- 4 weekly HbA1c + RBS

Gestational Diabetes
1st Visit

- Shown self blood glucose monitoring
- Bloods HbA1c, U&E's
- Dietetic Advice low fat/sugar high fibre
- Follow guidelines at appropriate gestation

N.B. Regime may vary slightly for each person
WANDA guidelines No:1. Version 2. Dated Jan 07.

Figure 17.2 Organisation of antenatal care for women with diabetes (provided by Dr Aresh Anwar, University Hospital, Coventry).

Table 17.4 Monitoring targets.

Fasting/pre-meal target	3.9–5.9 mmol/l
Post-prandial target (1 hour post meal)	<7.8 mmol/l

and frequent self-monitoring is required. The patient should visit a joint clinic in the outpatients department every 2 weeks. Patients are encouraged to check glucose levels post-prandially as well as fasting and pre-prandially, as better control of post-prandial hyperglycaemia can help achieve optimal control (Table 17.4).

Patients with type 2 diabetes who were previously on metformin alone will usually require insulin during pregnancy but in some cases, especially when they are needle-phobic they are managed safely with glibenclamide as it does not cross the placental barrier and is not associated with neonatal hypoglycaemia. Metformin has also been shown to be safe in pregnancy and can be used as a lone agent or with insulin.

The new rapid-acting insulin analogues such as aspart and lispro have been found to be particularly useful in pregnancy, and have advantages over soluble insulins. Whilst there is limited data on long-acting analogues, they have slowly become part of routine practice. Many units, however, continue to advocate the use of isophane in pregnancy. Patients who fail to achieve adequate glycaemic control despite multiple dose regimens should be considered for continuous subcutaneous insulin infusion (an insulin pump).

Managing diabetic complications during pregnancy (Table 17.5)

Women with pre-existing diabetic retinopathy may experience quite dramatic worsening of this complication with intensifying glycaemic control, especially if they have had poor control before. Therefore, regular examinations are required and they may require laser treatment. Women with hypertension and/or proteinuria are at great risk of accelerated hypertension and renal failure. In those patients with nephropathy and serum creatinine greater than 200 μmol/l, outcome is likely to be poor and the patient should be strongly advised not to get pregnant. Women with renal impairment can expect some deterioration of renal function

Table 17.5 Inter-relationship of diabetes and pregnancy.

Impact of diabetes on the baby
Increased miscarriage rate
Increased risk of congenital anomalies
Increased risk of macrosomia
Increased risk of stillbirth
Increased perinatal mortality

Impact of pregnancy on diabetes
Progression of retinopathy
Progression of nephropathy
Progression of neuropathy

Impact of diabetes on pregnancy
Increased risk of pre-eclampsia
Increased risk of polyhydramnios
Increased risk of Caesarean section

following the pregnancy. Hypertension in pregnancy should be managed using methyldopa, together with labetalol or amlodipine if needed. Those on angiotensin converting enzyme inhibitors should ideally be changed to the above agents before pregnancy. Statins should be stopped 3 months prior to planned conception.

Monitoring the foetus during pregnancy

The true value of foetal monitoring continues to be debated. A standard regime will start with a dating scan as soon as possible in pregnancy. This is normally followed by a more accurate dating scan at 11–12 weeks of gestation. There will then be a detailed scan at 20–21 weeks specifically examining the foetus for cardiac and central nervous system abnormalities. Serial scans assessing foetal growth normally start at 27 weeks with units varying the frequency with which they scan patients. A major risk to the foetus from diabetes is macrosomia (21% >4000 g versus 11% in general population) and a twofold increase in shoulder dystocia (7.9% versus around 3%). Assessment of foetal size, weight and health are important in determining the timing and mode of delivery.

There remains a high risk of unexplained late intrauterine death. The risk of this increases as the pregnancy progresses. As a consequence pregnancies of patients with diabetes are rarely allowed to progress to full term and patients are assessed for an appropriate delivery date from 38 weeks. Growth retardation is serious and requires specialist investigation.

Management in labour

Pregnant women with diabetes are usually admitted for a short period before the planned delivery or for a longer period when there are complications present. Monitoring of hyperglycaemia and also of the foetal heart rate is carried out. Although the aim is for a vaginal delivery in most cases, it is still by Caesarean section in many cases, at around 38 weeks gestation (Figure 17.3).

Figure 17.3 Proportion of pregnancies resulting in elective and emergency Caesarean sections (CS) and spontaneous vaginal delivery (SVD) based on Hospital Episode Statistics (HES) for England and Wales (2002/3) and the Confidential Enquiry into Maternal and Child Health (CEMACH) diabetes cohort.

Managing hyperglycaemia during labour

All obstetric units will have a regime for managing hyperglycaemia during labour. An example from the West Midlands Guidelines is given (Figures 17.4 and 17.5). Glucose and insulin are given by IV infusion and the rate of insulin infusion is adjusted to maintain blood glucose levels between 4–7 mmol/l. The IV insulin pump is maintained until the mother can start her normal meals. Many type 2 patients will not require insulin following delivery but doses should be reduced or adjusted according to plasma glucose levels.

The neonate

The most common neonatal complication is hypoglycaemia that still occurs in about one in five babies of mothers with diabetes. Hyperinsulinaemia results from placental transport of maternal insulin (endogenous or administered) that is surplus to the requirements of the infant. This is the cause of neonatal hypoglycaemia (and of foetal macrosomia, due to growth in a hyperinsulinaemic environment). Feeding should be encouraged as soon as possible (within 30 minutes) after delivery and every 2–3 hours thereafter. Neonatal blood glucose levels should be monitored regularly. If the level remains below 2.0 mmol/l on two occasions

Diabetic Intrapartum Care

Induction of Labour

- Aim to deliver at < 40 weeks gestation
  - decided on individual basis
- Inform Delivery Suite of admission
- Routine admission and induction procedure
- Continue present Insulin + diet reglme until in labour
- Intermittent FH auscultation/ CTG
- Prescribe:
  - Sliding scale Insulin + Dextrose regime
  - Glucagon (Type 1 diabetes)
  - Post delivery insulin regime
- Aim to keep glucoses between 4 – 7mmols/L (Commence Sliding Scale Insulin + Dextrose IV if not able to do so)
- Transfer to Delivery suite when in established labour or SROM

In established labour or for ARM

- Oral fluids for treatment of hypo's
- Commence IV sliding scale insulin + Dextrose as per protocol
- Continuous CTG.
- 2 – 4 hourly cervical assessment for early diagnosis of obstructed labour

Syntocinon regime to be given via a separate venflon

- Low threshold for felal blood sampling
- Be aware of shoulder dystocia and risk of fetal macrosomia
- Accurate documentation of partogram of maternal observations, fetal heart rate and progress of labour/ timing of interventions
- Senior obstetric Involvement

For L.S.C.S.

- Admit day before
- Routine admission + CTG
- Routine bloods. FBC. Group and Save + pre - op procedure
- Inform Delivery Suite of her admission.
- **DO NOT ALLOW TO GO HOME**
- Prescribe:
  - Sliding scale insulin + Dextrose
  - Post delivery insulin regime
  - Glucagon 1 mg (Type 1 diabetics)
- **N.B.M. from midnight.**
- Treat hypoglycaemia with Dextrose Tabs x 3 or Glucogel then transfer to delivery suite for Sliding scale Insulin + Dextrose

Following morning

- Omit morning dose of insulin.
- Listen to the fetal heart.
- Transfer to Delivery suite 07.00 - 08.00 hrs
- Commence IV Sliding scale Insulin + Dextrose as per protocol

Gestational Diabetes
- Stop infusion once placenta delivered

When and how to shop a sliding scale insulin post delivery

Pre pregnancy Diabetes
- Ensure patient is eating and drinking normally
- Give insulin when next due. (Regime in notes)
- Provide meal or snack.
- Stop insulin + Dextrose after 30 mins

N.B. Regime may vary slightly for each person, please check notes

WANDA. guidelines No:2. Version 2. Dated Jan 07.

Figure 17.4 Management of blood glucose during delivery (provided by Dr Aresh Anwar, University Hospital, Coventry).

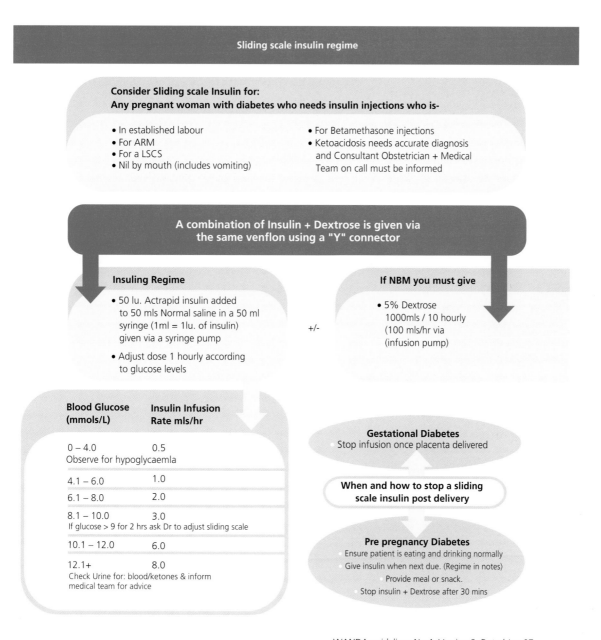

WANDA guidelines No:4. Version 2. Dated Jan 07.

Figure 17.5 Insulin sliding scale for use during delivery (provided by Dr Aresh Anwar, University Hospital, Coventry).

despite adequate feeding (or if feeding is ineffective) then tube feeding or intravenous dextrose should be considered. Respiratory distress syndrome is a complication if the baby is delivered prematurely, particularly when the mother has had poor glycaemic control. Occasionally, other complications such as polycythaemia and hypocalcaemia may occur. Macrosomia contributes significantly to both maternal and neonatal morbidity.

Breastfeeding is encouraged just as in non-diabetic mothers and the mother's diet is increased by about 50 g of carbohydrate daily. Breastfeeding mothers should not use oral hypoglycaemic agents. Use of metformin during breastfeeding is not recommended by the manufacturers.

Postnatal follow up of gestational diabetes

Following the postnatal checks a glucose tolerance test is arranged about 6–8 weeks after delivery. A majority return to normal glucose tolerance; however, these women do have an increased risk of developing type 2 diabetes over the next 5 years. Even if the glucose tolerance test is normal an annual check of fasting blood glucose is advised and they are advised to continue with a healthy life-style. They should also be told that they are virtually certain to have gestational diabetes in future pregnancies. Those diagnosed to have persistent diabetes following the postnatal glucose tolerance test

Postnatal care for diabetes

Type 1 + 2 diabetes

- Close monitoring of glucose levels
- Type 2 patients previously on oral hypoglycaemic agents should remain on insulin if wanting to breastfeed
  - (metformin used in some units in overweight patients)
- If breastfeeding increase carbohydrate intake + insulin may need to be reduced by as much as 20%
- Oberve and treat hypoglycaemia (See flowchart)
- Review by the Diabetes Specialist midwife or Medical Team

Gestational diabetes

- Blood glucose measurements for 24–48 hrs initially to ensure levels are returning back to normal
- OGTT at 6–8 weeks post delivery.
- All women are informed of the risks of developing Type 2 diabetes later in life (Preventative measures i.e. diet, exercise, ideal weight plus yearly follow ups with their GP)

All women
Normal postnatal care
- Do not allow 6 hr discharge
- Daily inspection of wounds for infection and treat promptly
- Breastfeeding encouraged
- Discussion of future pregnancy plans and advice
- Contraceptive advice prior to discharge
- Document management plan at home and FU arrangements

Care of the baby
- Breastfeeding encouraged
- Feed within 1hr of age then 3 hrly
- At risk of hypoglycaemla, regular glucose measurements (follow guidelines for baby at risk of hypoglycaemla)
- Keep with mother unless specific indication for
- Neonatal unit admission, see guideline No. 7
- Observe for signs of jaundice

WANDA guidelines No:5. Version 2. Dated Jan 07.

Figure 17.6 Postnatal care guidelines for all types of diabetes in pregnancy (provided by Dr Aresh Anwar, University Hospital, Coventry).

are treated like other patients with type 2 diabetes. Figure 17.6 summarises postpartum care for mothers and babies following a diabetic pregnancy.

Summary

Pregnancy places a physiological strain on maternal glucose tolerance, precipitating gestational diabetes in those at risk and threatening to destabilise pre-existing diabetes. In either scenario, a substantially increased risk of complicated pregnancy justifies proactive, coordinated management to improve maternal and neonatal outcomes. This approach should commence before pregnancy through preconceptual interventions including tightening of glycaemic control, withdrawal of potentially teratogenic medications, and prescription of high dose folic acid. The majority of patients affected will require insulin during pregnancy to achieve optimal glycaemic targets. The newer rapid-acting insulin analogues may be particularly useful in this setting. Delivery of the infant may restore previous glucose tolerance in the mother but close monitoring is required to detect neonatal hypoglycaemia. For those with gestational diabetes diagnosed during the pregnancy, follow-up is essential to confirm resolution and to screen for future incident diabetes. Patient education is important at all stages to optimise outcomes.

Further reading

Confidential Enquiry into Maternal and Child Health: *Pregnancy in Women with Type 1 and Type 2 Diabetes in 2002–03, England, Wales and Northern Ireland*. CEMACH, London, 2005.

Getahun D, Nath C, Ananth CV, *et al.* Gestational diabetes in the United States: temporal trends 1989 through 2004. *Am J Obstet Gynecol.* 2008;**198**: 525.e1–5.

National Institute of Health and Clinical Excellence. *Diabetes in pregnancy*. Clinical guideline No 63. March 2008.

Guideline Development Group, NICE and Mugglestone, M. Management of diabetes from preconception to the postnatal period: summary of NICE guidance. *BMJ* 2008;**336**(7646):714–717.

Zhang X, Decker A, Platt RW, Kramer MS. How big is too big? The perinatal consequences of fetal macrosomia. *Am J Obstet Gynecol.* 2008;**198**: 517.e1–6.

CHAPTER 18

Organisation of Diabetes Care in General Practice

Tim Holt[1] and Sudhesh Kumar[2]

[1]Health Sciences Research Institute, Warwick Medical School, University of Warwick, Coventry, UK
[2]Clinical Sciences Research Institute, Warwick Medical School, University of Warwick; and WISDEM, University Hospital, Coventry, UK

OVERVIEW

- Quality diabetes care requires well-developed organisational infrastructure

- The Diabetes Register is central both for surveillance and audit

- Annual reviews should be offered to all patients but most will require more frequent contact to monitor progress towards targets, address emerging problems, and screen for early complications

- Monitoring quality of care may be a practice-based activity or may occur at a higher level through integrated information technology, depending on the health care setting

- Measuring quality of care should include not only numerical indices that are electronically coded, but also the qualitative aspects, including access, continuity and patient satisfaction

Introduction

The majority of diabetes care, particularly for type 2 patients, can be provided by non-specialist clinicians who have ready access to specialist advice. The increasing prevalence of type 2 diabetes makes this the most effective use of resources, saving specialist expertise for when it is really required. Primary care clinicians need to maintain and develop their expertise within a multidisciplinary team of professionals. Structured care programmes involving regular surveillance, and clearly understood referral pathways to secondary care are essential components of this infrastructure.

Diabetes Register

Central to any surveillance programme is the Diabetes Register. Ideally, everyone with diabetes should be recorded on the Diabetes Register of one care provider. This provider can then identify all the patients with diabetes for whom the team is responsible. In this way, it is clear to everyone who is responsible for whose care. In the UK this is achieved through registration in general practice, and all NHS patients have a NHS number that is their 'unique identifier'. The

general practitioners manage the majority of diabetes surveillance, and for patients under hospital follow-up (including most children) they nevertheless audit the control parameters as a back-up to hospital-based audits. This means that the primary care diabetes registers include everyone known to have diabetes in the community.

> Whilst patients increasingly take and share responsibility for treatment decisions and follow up, health care providers must recognise their own corporate responsibility for ensuring high quality care to all their registered patients

Quality of the Diabetes Register

Organisation of care revolves around the register, but we should not forget about those in the community who are missing from it (see the overlapping but non-identical circles in Figure 18.1). No diabetes register is perfect, and it is likely to not only miss a significant number of cases (estimated 1% of the UK population) but also to include patients who on more rigorous testing would not fulfil the diagnostic criteria. Mechanisms for improving and maintaining the quality of the diabetes register should be built into the daily processes of routine care, to ensure as close an overlap as possible. These include active case finding for undiagnosed patients, adherence to recommended criteria for diagnosis, and removal of patients from the register that have moved out of the area and registered for care elsewhere.

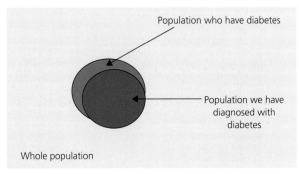

Figure 18.1 A high quality diabetes register ensures the population with diabetes is identified as accurately as possible so that the circles overlap closely.

ABC of Diabetes, 6th edition. By T. Holt and S. Kumar.
Published 2010 by Blackwell Publishing.

88

In most economically developed countries the Register will take the form of an electronic database. But whatever form it takes, two requirements are essential:

- The Register can identify everyone known to have diabetes
- Searches can be undertaken to identify individuals who are due surveillance or whose results are out of target

In the UK, surveillance for complications takes place predominantly in primary care. Chapter 11 describes the regular surveillance procedures recommended as part of structured care (Boxes 18.1 and 18.2).

Box 18.1 Overall aim of diabetes care

- To achieve a quality of life and life-expectancy similar to that of the general population
- To reduce the symptoms and the complications of diabetes whilst enjoying a flexible life-style
- To treat those with diabetes individually and involve them in all aspects of their care, empowering them with the knowledge and skills to feel in control of their diabetes

Box 18.2 Cornerstones of diabetes care organisation

- Identification of those at risk
- Reduction of both diabetes and cardiovascular risk in the 'at-risk' population
- Early detection of diabetes
- Comprehensive education and life-style advice tailored to the individual and carers
- Prescribed medication and referral within an extended team of professionals
- Access to information and help during and between regular reviews
- Regular surveillance for complications
- Early, active intervention for developing complications

Case finding for diabetes

Screening the whole population for diabetes is inefficient and not currently recommended, but *case finding* by targeting at-risk groups (Box 18.3) is worthwhile.

Box 18.3 Groups who justify regular testing for diabetes

- Known cardiovascular disease, hypertension, or hyperlipidaemia
- Impaired glucose tolerance or impaired fasting glycaemia
- Metabolic syndrome characteristics
- Family history of type 2 diabetes
- Ethnicity: South Asian, Afro-Caribbean, American Indian, Pacific Islanders
- History of gestational diabetes

- Drug therapy, e.g. corticosteroids
- Polycystic ovaries plus obesity
- Chronic mental illness

How often should we test?

Generally speaking at least every 3 years. However, people with impaired glucose tolerance (IGT), impaired fasting glycaemia (IFG) or a history of gestational diabetes require testing annually (see below) and should be advised to return sooner if diabetes symptoms develop in the meantime.

Follow-up of borderline random blood glucose results

All random glucose measurements ≥ 6.1 justify follow-up testing by fasting plasma glucose (FPG) and HbA1c. Before arranging this, find out:

1 Does the patient have any symptoms of diabetes (thirst, polyuria, unexplained weight loss)?
2 Was the original blood glucose test actually random or fasting (this may be unclear in the notes)?

Diabetes needs then to be established or excluded in the way described in Chapter 1. Clinical suspicion of diabetes may justify repeated testing at intervals determined by perceived risk.

Follow-up of gestational diabetes

Those with a history of gestational diabetes are at raised life-long risk of type 2 diabetes. Where glucose tolerance has returned to normal after delivery, a fasting plasma glucose should be offered annually

Organising care following the diagnosis

Explaining the diagnosis to the patient

The quality of explanation and information given to the newly diagnosed patient is an important factor in long-term concordance and in promoting self-efficacy, and so is worth the time investment. Patients sometimes have specific beliefs about the cause of diabetes or why it has happened to them. These are worth discussing. From an organisational point of view the time required to cover these areas needs protecting.

Initial assessment
Measurements
At the first assessment following the diagnosis the following measurements should be taken:

- Weight
- Body mass index
- Height
- Waist circumference
- Blood pressure
- Urine for microalbumin

Monitoring and surveillance arrangements

- Arrange retinopathy screening
- Arrange blood test for
  - Baseline HbA1c (unless already done in the past 3 months)
  - Urea and electrolytes and estimated glomerular filtration rate (e-GFR)
  - Liver function tests
  - Baseline fasting lipids including total serum cholesterol, HDL cholesterol, LDL cholesterol and triglycerides

The majority of patients presenting will have type 2 diabetes and be at least overweight at diagnosis. If the patient has a normal body mass index, or is losing weight, this should be noted and drawn to the attention of a clinician responsible for insulin initiation. Such patients may be insulin-deficient and might need insulin early on in the course of their treatment.

Treatment pathways are discussed in Chapters 6 and 8, and surveillance in Chapter 11.

Self-monitoring

All insulin-dependent patients (type 1 and type 2) should be taught how to self-monitor, as well as other selected groups (see Chapter 10). For type 2 patients this should occur before insulin is commenced. Test strips can be prescribed in boxes of 50. The volume of blood required is very small, and can be taken from the fingers, forearm, upper arm, thigh or calf. If it is taken at the fingers, the finger edge rather than the central pulp is preferable, to avoid long-term loss of sensation. This is particularly important for those with low vision or those at risk of it. All patients who self-monitor should be prescribed a sharps bin and this should be left on the 'Repeat' screen so that it can be easily reordered.

Frequency of self-monitoring

Usage of strips will vary between patients and treatment regimens. Those needing to monitor most frequently are patients on flexible basal bolus regimens, particularly when they are carbohydrate counting and adjusting insulin doses frequently (see section on DAFNE, page 44). Such an approach is only safe if self-monitoring is frequent *and* if the patient is adequately skilled at interpreting and responding to variation in glucose measurements. Type 2 patients taking once daily long-acting insulin will have less frequent need for self-monitoring but should still be taught it, as this will help to titrate the dose during the first few weeks of therapy and to adjust it thereafter.

Self-monitoring in patients not on insulin

Type 2 patients not taking insulin benefit much less from self-monitoring, which needs to be justified in the individual. For those who *are* self-monitoring, frequency should be kept to once or twice a week, and fasting readings are generally more beneficial in such patients as a marker of control than random measurements. However, there is increasing interest in post-prandial rises in blood glucose as an independent risk factor for vascular complications.

The International Diabetes Federation have established a guideline committee to address this issue. Well-controlled HbA1c remains the prime treatment target for glycaemic control. The situation changes if the patient later starts insulin, as avoidance of hypoglycaemia then becomes a more important issue. Patients taking sulphonylureas who drive may need to monitor before starting a journey.

Follow-up

After the initial assessment, a follow-up appointment should be made at an appropriate interval. For most type 2 patients, treatment decisions will need to be reviewed after 2–3 months. Regular reviews during this period are a good idea to answer questions, build confidence, reinforce successful changes, and detect the occasional patient with deteriorating insulin deficiency. Generally, type 2 patients out of target for HbA1c (<7.0% or 53 mmol/mol) should be reviewed with repeat HbA1c every 3 months after each change in treatment until in target and then 6-monthly thereafter.

Starting insulin in general practice

Type 1 patients, who present acutely, should be referred without delay to secondary care services. They may or may not need hospital admission, but are at risk of ketoacidosis and require close monitoring, education, and frequent follow-up in the early stages. This is best carried out under the supervision of a specialist team including Diabetes Specialist Nurses. Management of type 2 patients requiring insulin is discussed in Chapters 6 and 8.

Assessing the quality of diabetes care

Diabetes Audit and Research in Tayside Scotland (DARTS)

In addition to the practice-based diabetes register, combined registers involving multiple practices may be linked together for research or audit purposes. This first occurred in the UK in 1997 in Tayside, with the DARTS project. Linkage of records from primary and secondary care sources improved the detection of diabetes cases, and data from the University of Dundee Medicines Monitoring Unit (MEMO) enabled prescribing data to be matched to clinical outcomes at an individual level using anonymised identifiers. Research outcomes from this project included the finding that self-monitoring (based on usage of testing strips) was uncommon in both type 1 and type 2 patients, but that HbA1c levels were lower in type 1 patients who self-monitored frequently (Evans *et al.* 1999).

The Quality and Outcomes Framework

One of the advantages of a searchable diabetes register is the ease with which regular audit on the quality of care may be carried out. In the United Kingdom, this facility is provided through the 'Quality and Outcomes Framework', introduced in April 2004 (Figure 18.2). General Practitioners are given payments according to the proportion of patients achieving specified quality standards at the end of the year. Each audit standard attracts payment

Figure 18.2 Population manager software at the practice of one of the editors, enabling the practice team to monitor progress towards treatment targets, and listing the 'points' available for each indicator. The annual influenza immunisation programme is yet to start. Work is required on the proportion of patients with albuminuria who are prescribed ACE inhibitors or A2RB agents (currently only 76% against a target of 80%). Individuals outside any of the targets are easily identifiable through drop down lists and their medical records can then be browsed directly. Other UK based Clinical software systems provide similar facilities.

'points', whose value relates to the importance of the parameter as a determinant of outcomes and its achievability. Regular practice meetings identify areas of care that are falling short of the standards specified. The patients currently out of target for each parameter can be readily identified through a drop-down box accessed by clicking on the appropriate page. A system of alert messages identifies which parameters are out of target each time a patient's notes are opened. The QOF relies on a system of integrated practice-based software linked to the local laboratory, and on the consistent electronic coding of the necessary parameters. Diabetes currently accounts for 93 of the 655 'points' available for clinical care, reflecting the priority this condition is given.

Payment by results: pros and cons

The benefits for patient care resulting from the QOF are evident using intermediate outcome measures such as blood pressure and glycaemic control. It will take longer to demonstrate an impact on mortality and serious morbidity. Many in primary care welcome the QOF – general practitioners generally feel they are being paid appropriately for the evidence-based management of serious chronic disease, and patient advocacy groups recognise the potential benefits arising from financial incentives. However, there are negative aspects. There may be adverse effects on clinician-patient relationships, as primary care has become extremely target-driven, and the aspects of care that are not easily measured may be out-prioritised. Clinicians may become preoccupied with numerical data and neglect the qualitative aspects of care that patients value. Another criticism is that the same targets are applied to heterogenous sub-groups of patients, failing to recognise individual needs, and that the elderly may be treated too aggressively. The QOF is reviewed annually to examine such effects and changes are made based on wide consultation with stake holding bodies including those representing patients and their carers.

Significant events

Care may be improved by team discussion of 'significant events' where issues or problems have arisen that might have been better dealt with. This should be a regular activity. It is based on individual cases, and should supplement (and not simply replace) a regular programme of audit involving the entire population with diabetes under the team's care. Possible significant events that may be worth examining are suggested in Box 18.4 but there are many other possibilities.

Box 18.4 **Cases worth examining and discussing among the team**

- **A type 2 patient presenting with HbA1c >12% (108 mmol/mol) at diagnosis:** This suggests late presentation (unless the clinical picture is that of insulin deficiency, with weight loss). Looking back through the records over 5 years, were previous borderline or raised blood glucose levels recorded but not followed up? Were possible diabetes symptoms reported but not investigated with diabetes in mind? Was the patient identifiably at risk but not included in active case finding?

- **A patient requiring amputation:** This is a serious event that may reflect a failure of preventive care. Was everything done to minimise the risk of this complication? Was the protocol for surveillance followed and is it understood by the entire team? Were risk factors identified and actively managed? Are the indications and mechanisms for referral to secondary care widely understood within the practice?

- **A patient not requesting important medication:** Are the practice's mechanisms for access to repeat prescriptions and consultations robust? Are there difficulties in accessing help? Does the patient understand the importance of regular review? If not, why not?

Patient satisfaction and feedback

Patients should be offered opportunities to feed back and comment on the quality of care provided by the team. This should involve both active and passive strategies:

- Patient satisfaction surveys, carried out periodically, to actively seek feedback
- Suggestions box
- Complaints procedure
- Patient support groups feeding back to the practice team

Summary

Well-developed organisational infrastructure is essential to high-quality diabetes care. Multidisciplinary teamwork requires clearly understood processes and referral pathways, providing good communication and clear allocation of clinical and administrative responsibilities. These processes should cover the early detection and diagnosis of diabetes, through which individuals enter the diabetes register; the initial assessment and education of the patient; regular surveillance, follow-up and cross-referral within the extended team; and availability of interventions for the effective prevention and treatment of complications.

Further reading

Morris AD, Boyle DIR, MacAlpine R, *et al*. The diabetes audit and research in Tayside Scotland (DARTS) study: electronic record linkage to create a diabetes register. *BMJ* 1997;**315**:524–8.

Evans JMM, Newton RW, Ruta DA, MacDonald TM, Stevenson RJ, and Morris AD. Frequency of blood glucose monitoring in relation to glycaemic control: observational study with diabetes database. *BMJ* 1999;**319**:83–6.

http://www.qof.ic.nhs.uk/

CHAPTER 19

New and Emerging Therapies for Diabetes

Tim Holt[1] and Sudhesh Kumar[2]

[1]Health Sciences Research Institute, Warwick Medical School, University of Warwick, Coventry, UK
[2]Clinical Sciences Research Institute, Warwick Medical School, University of Warwick; and WISDEM, University Hospital, Coventry, UK

OVERVIEW

- Modern management of both hyperglycaemia and obesity is still inadequate for a substantial proportion of patients

- Progressive beta cell failure is particularly difficult to treat in overweight patients who are insulin-resistant

- Emerging approaches involve new physiological pathways including the incretin system and the cannabinoid receptors, but there are still problems

- Future progress is likely to involve not only novel drug classes but also non-pharmacological approaches including islet cell transplantation and the artificial pancreas

---

Introduction

Despite the best efforts of the patient and supporting clinicians, it is not always possible to control diabetes adequately, prevent the progression of the condition or treat its devastating complications. Part of the problem may be related to the heterogeneity of diabetes that we currently ignore in our empirical approach to the management of hyperglycaemia. In the future, personalised therapy based on the underlying causes may help improve outcomes. The last few years have seen intense activity in the pharmaceutical and biotechnology industries to develop more varied modalities of treatment for controlling hyperglycaemia.

Key limitations of current therapeutic approaches

There are a number of problems associated with current therapy. First, it should be recognised that major limitations exist in our delivery of diabetes care and in empowering patients to self-manage their condition. Improvements here will help get better outcomes from our existing therapies. Some features of type 2 diabetes in particular, make it difficult to manage with our existing therapies. The most important problems are:

- **Beta cell failure.** Prevention of beta cell destruction could potentially prevent type 1 diabetes in susceptible individuals and

significantly reduce the risk of progression of type 2 diabetes and the need for insulin

- **Obesity.** One problem with a number of our therapies for diabetes is weight gain. This is not appreciated by patients and with obesity comes many other risk factors because of the known relationship between obesity, blood pressure and dyslipidaemia

- **Hypoglycaemia.** This is a feared complication of diabetes and a major impediment to improving glycaemic control. Hypoglycaemia can blight an individual's life and it is important to try and avoid this

- **Control of post-prandial hyperglycaemia.** Recently there has been more attention given to post-prandial hyperglycaemia because of recognition of its relationship to vascular disease risk. Control of post-prandial hyperglycaemia is important in order to get better control of overall hyperglycaemia

- **Insulin resistance.** Type 2 is in part due to defects in insulin action and in those with marked insulin defects this means large doses of insulin and difficulty in achieving tight glucose control

- **Other side effects.** There are side effects related to various drugs available today that limit therapy, for example gastrointestinal side effects with metformin and alpha-glycosidase inhibitors, fluid retention and osteopenia with thiazolidinediones (glitazones) and hypoglycaemia and weight gain for sulphonylureas

Many of the following groups of newer drugs are advantageous in terms of one or more of the above aspects. However, one limitation of newer therapies is that we do not yet have evidence of long-term benefits through reduction of complications or long-term safety. Therefore, the potential for improvement in hyperglycaemia and lack of side effects must be placed in the above context.

Pramlintide

Pramlintide is an antidiabetic agent that mimics the activity of the hormone amylin which is co-secreted along with insulin from the pancreatic islets. It is available in the United States for mealtime control of hyperglycaemia as an addition to insulin therapy. It acts mainly by altering the rate of gastric emptying, and also reducing the rise of glucagon levels following meals. It is given as a separate injection to insulin and can produce additional improvement in glucose control. It is currently not available in the UK.

ABC of Diabetes, 6th edition. By T. Holt and S. Kumar.
Published 2010 by Blackwell Publishing.

Incretins and other hormone-based therapies

Incretins are endogenous gut hormones including glucagon-like peptide-1 (GLP-1) and glucose-dependant insulinotrophic polypeptide (GIP). They have useful insulin-releasing and other glucose-regulatory actions. Preparations of GLP-1 analogues or modified formulations of this peptide (GLP-1 mimetics) have been developed for the treatment of type 2 diabetes. Another class of drugs is based on an understanding of how these endogenous peptides are degraded in the body. Enzymes called dipeptidyl peptidase IV (DPP4) rapidly degrade endogenous GLP-1. Oral agents have been developed that inhibit DPP4 and therefore prolong the activity of endogenous GLP-1.

Examples of the former approach include Exenatide and Liraglutide, and there are numerous others in developments. An example of the latter are a new class of drugs called DDP4 inhibitors. Sitagliptin and Vildagliptin are currently available in the UK and numerous others are in development.

GLP-1

Glucagon-like peptide-1 has the potential to improve glucose metabolism through a variety of different actions as shown in Figure 19.1. Perhaps the most exciting is the suggested potential to improve beta cell insulin biosynthesis. They also inhibit secretion of glucagon, a somewhat neglected hormone in diabetes thus far. Figure 19.2 shows the impairment of the normal incretin response in patients with type 2 diabetes. The incretin Exenatide is currently available in many countries and a long-acting preparation is also in development. It is started at a dose of 5 mg twice daily by subcutaneous injection as the initiation of therapies is often associated with nausea. The dose is then increased to 10 mg twice daily. Use of GLP-1 agonists do not preclude patients from driving. This is therefore particularly useful in patients whose occupation depends on driving public service vehicles. These patients would otherwise lose their livelihood if they start insulin. However, if adequate glycaemic control is not achieved with a GLP-1 agonist then it is important to advise the patient that insulin is necessary. When GLP-1 agonists are added to other oral agents a further 1% (11 mmol/mol) reduction or so in HbA1c can be expected, although some patients may achieve more or less than this. A useful additional effect is weight loss, which is particularly useful in overweight or obese type 2 patients. Excess risk of pancreatitis has been observed in post-marketing studies although the absolute number of events is very small. It is, however, wise to avoid it in patients who may be otherwise at risk of pancreatitis. It is currently not advisable to use this along with insulin, as combination therapy has been shown to result in much higher rates of hypoglycaemia. If prescribed with sulphonylureas it is important that should hypoglycaemia occur, the dose of sulphonylurea is reduced. Liraglutide is a more recently introduced GLP-1 analogue that is given as a single daily dose.

DDP4 Inhibitors

As oral agents these are a useful addition to metformin or sulphonylureas as they appear to be relatively well tolerated with no major side effects that have come to light so far. Sitagliptin was the first to become available in the UK and is initially prescribed at a dose of 100 mg daily. Vildagliptin is available at a dose of 50 mg daily. They generally produce reductions of HbA1c between 0.7 and 1% (7.7–11 mmol/mol) , do not produce hypoglycaemia on their own and are weight-neutral. These drugs are useful additional therapy as they may produce further reduction in hyperglycaemia. As with GLP-1 agonist therapy, no long-term outcome data are available with this class of drugs.

Obesity

Life-style modification is difficult once patients have type 2 diabetes. The disease itself and the drugs often used by patients with diabetes mean that progressive weight gain often occurs. Reduction in weight using drug therapy brings with it benefits in terms of

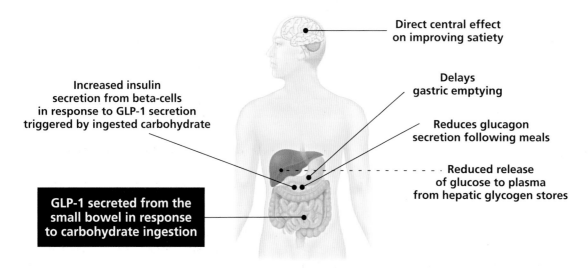

Figure 19.1 Multiple effects of the incretin GLP-1 on glucose regulation.

The Incretin Effect: Response to Oral vs IV Glucose

Mean ± SE; N = 6; *$P \leq .05$; 0_1–0_2 = glucose infusion time.

The Incretin Effect: Is Reduced in Patients With Type 2 Diabetes

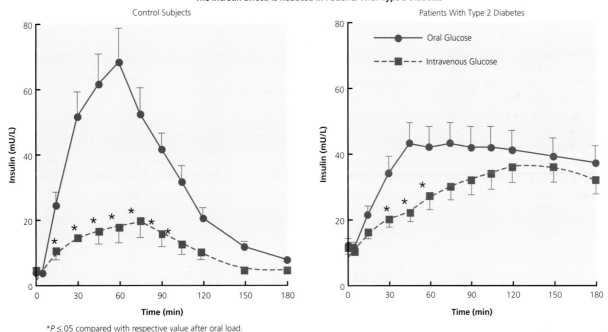

*$P \leq .05$ compared with respective value after oral load.

Figure 19.2 Endogenous insulin secretion (measured by C-peptide) responds more to oral than to intravenous glucose challenge due to the incretin effect. This effect is impaired in type 2 diabetes. Reproduced with kind permission from Springer Science+Business Media. Nauck M. *Diabetologia* 1986;**29**:46–52.

concomitant improvements in glycaemia although these are often modest to the extent of about 0.5% (5.5 mmol/mol) of HbA1c reduction with orlistat and sibutramine. These are useful additions to therapy for obese patients with type 2 diabetes. However, these drugs are ineffective or their use is contra-indicated in many patients with obesity and diabetes. Therefore, there is a need for newer agents for obesity, especially if they have additional effects or added value in terms of improvement of associated risk factors including diabetes.

Endocannabinoid system and CB1 receptor antagonists

Several CB1 antagonists are in development and Rimonabant was available in many countries before it was withdrawn because of concerns over adverse effects. Rimonabant crosses the blood brain barrier and inhibits CB1 receptors in the hypothalamus leading to reduction in appetite and improvement in satiety. They also have been shown to have direct effect on adipose tissue in the visceral fat depot. This is reflected in weight loss and useful reduction in waist circumference, which is associated with reduction in HbA1c of about 0.7% (7.7 mmol/mol). There is also significant improvement in HDL cholesterol and reduction in triglyceride and expected reductions in blood pressure with the weight loss.

The major disadvantage that was identified with Rimonabant is the tendency to cause mood disorders. Some other drugs in the same class are no longer being developed following withdrawal of Rimonabant due to this concern.

Other anti-obesity drugs

Glucocorticoid hormone pathways are being explored to produce new compounds that either inhibit their action or modulate their metabolism. 11β Hydroxysteroid dehydrogenase (11βHSD) type 1 enzyme inhibitors have potential to reverse central obesity and attendant complications. They are currently being subjected to trials. Adipose tissue also secretes a number of peptides that have been recently recognised. Potential new therapies based on understanding of adipose tissue biology are also being developed.

The future

Protein kinase C (PKC) inhibitors

Reducing the risk of complications in patients with diabetes is achieved mainly through control of blood glucose, blood pressure and dyslipidaemia. Clearly, this should be pursued with vigour to obtain the best control that can be achieved in the patient. Despite this, there are numerous patients whose glycaemic control remains poor. In such patients there is potential for drug therapy to prevent the hyperglycaemia-induced damage on tissues that cause the complications. One such agent is a protein kinase C (PKC) inhibitor that has been developed recently. At the moment ruboxistaurin remains in phase 3 development as it requires further data to establish efficacy, although its safety appears to be quite good over a 3-year period.

Artificial pancreas

Improvements in the technology of continuous monitoring and insulin delivery raise the prospect of a future 'artificial pancreas' through closure of the feedback loop between glucose measurements and insulin infusion rates. Work on such devices is actively under way, but at present the monitoring technology is still not quite accurate enough for use in everyday situations. It is likely that this approach will be developed initially in intensively controlled hospital settings before the same principle can be used in portable devices.

Pancreas and islet cell transplantation

Whole organ pancreas transplantation is possible and has been particularly useful in patients also requiring kidney transplantation, as there is already a need for immunosuppressive therapy in such cases. Avoidance of the drawbacks of whole organ donation is potentially possible by transplanting human islets of Langerhans, but this has proven extremely difficult due to aggressive, largely cell-mediated rejection responses in the host. These rejection mechanisms are more difficult to control than those following transplantation of heart, liver or kidney, for reasons that are still not well understood. Advances in this area will require these immunological barriers to be overcome, or may result from future stem cell technology.

Further reading

Deacon CF. Incretin-based treatment of type 2 diabetes: glucagon-like peptide-1 receptor agonists and dipeptidyl peptidase-4 inhibitors. *Diabetes Obes Metab* 2007;**9**(s1):23–31.

Hovorka R. Continuous glucose monitoring and closed loop systems. *Diabet Med* 2005;**23**:1–12.

Jung PJ, Merrell RC. Update on pancreatic islet cell transplantation. *Semin Surgical Oncol* 2006;**6**:122–5.

Seaberg RM, Smukler SR, Kieffer TJ, *et al.* Clonal identification of multipotent precursors from adult mouse pancreas that generate neural and pancreatic lineages. *Nat Biotechnol* 2004;**22**:1115–24.

CHAPTER 20

Support for People Living with Diabetes

Tim Holt[1] and Sudhesh Kumar[2]

[1]Health Sciences Research Institute, Warwick Medical School, University of Warwick, Coventry, UK
[2]Clinical Sciences Research Institute, Warwick Medical School, University of Warwick; and WISDEM, University Hospital, Coventry, UK

OVERVIEW

- Living with diabetes may be a personal issue, or may be an experience shared with an expanding global community
- Accessing practical advice and support to help live with diabetes has become much easier due to web-based resources
- A wide range of materials is available for patients, their carers and health professionals, for advice, education and advocacy
- Support organisations also provide for those with no Internet access, and those with physical barriers such as sensory impairments

---

Introduction

A huge amount of help is available for people with diabetes, ranging from local groups offering individual support to international bodies advising patients, their carers and their health professionals (Figure 20.1). Advice and information needs to be tailored to the individual's needs and abilities, but provided sufficient time is taken most patients can understand the basic principles of diabetes care, and of course many become 'experts'. The Alphabet strategy, discussed earlier in this book, is as much about educating patients as it is about guiding clinicians on management. The Alphabet team have developed a range of readily accessible information sheets to assist in patient education (Figure 20.2). This gets the message across much more effectively than words alone.

Patient support organisations

For some, diabetes is a personal issue managed within a limited network of friends, family and health professionals, whilst for others this network extends to the wider community and beyond. Diabetes can affect anyone at almost any age. Many find amongst this diversity a common thread of shared experience. For others it is a very individual and private experience. Despite increasing public awareness of their needs, some people with diabetes may still feel isolated, stigmatised, discriminated against, or otherwise in need

---

ABC of Diabetes, 6th edition. By T. Holt and S. Kumar.
Published 2010 by Blackwell Publishing.

of support and advocacy. Others may wish to share their success at overcoming personal goals. For all types of people and for all those caring for them in any capacity, help is widely available. Over the last 20 years the accessibility of health information has blurred the distinction between advice aimed at patients and that aimed towards health professionals, so that many of the organisations provide for all through a common point of access.

The websites of some major organisations are included in the Further Reading section at the end of the chapter. Familiarity with these resources is important for clinicians, who need to be able to advise patients on the most appropriate web resources, as many are available that are misleading. They may also need to direct patients to locally relevant information that is not always as clearly signposted.

Diabetes UK

This is the major charity representing and supporting people with diabetes and their carers in the UK.

Diabetes UK has nearly 400 volunteer support groups all over the UK to provide peer support at a local as well as national level. Fundraising, campaigning, awareness raising and mutual support and advocacy are central activities, often taking place in social settings. The charity can help with practical issues such as finding affordable health insurance that does not discriminate unfairly towards those with diabetes. The charity awards a prize for those who have lived with diabetes for over 50 years, an increasing number annually.

Balance, a magazine for people with diabetes is published bi-monthly and there are also regular e-newsletters keeping people up to date with what is going on in diabetes care. Many of the resources are available in different languages and there is also CD- and audiotape-based information for those with visual impairment.

Diabetes UK also provides support for health professionals through policy statements, conferences, training materials, updates, and research funding. It influences national policy as the major UK stake holder representing users of diabetes services and is consulted on policy development including that of the National Institute of Health and Clinical Excellence (NICE). It holds an Annual Professional Conference and publishes a monthly professional journal *Diabetic Medicine*. This journal is available free to those in the developing world through the World Health Organization's

Figure 20.1 Patient information leaflets from the Alphabet team.

Figure 20.2 Seventy years on insulin: presenting in 1938 as a seven year old with thirst and weight loss, this patient was started on insulin and rapidly regained her health. Pictured here with her current GP, Dr Tim Holt.

HINARI programme. In addition, *Diabetes Update* is a quarterly journal on the latest news in diabetes.

The International Diabetes Federation (IDF)

The IDF applies similar principles to the worldwide community involved with diabetes, including patients, their carers and health professionals, and the research community. Their mission is 'to promote diabetes care, prevention and a cure worldwide'. They serve as an umbrella for national diabetes organisations all over the world. As well as its role in patient advocacy and education, the IDF has a strong academic role, e.g. producing the IDF definition of the metabolic syndrome discussed in Chapter 4, which has become widely adopted.

The IDF's quarterly publication *Diabetes Voice* is published in English, French and Spanish, and covers all aspects of diabetes care, education, prevention, research and practical aspects of living with diabetes.

The American Diabetes Association

Whilst aimed at an American readership, the ADA's website contains lots of useful links that will be of interest to people in all countries, including those wishing to keep up with the latest research in diabetes. They also provide useful dietary advice (see Box 20.1) and recipes.

Box 20.1 Practical advice on healthy eating from the American Diabetes Association website

- Eat lots of vegetables and fruits. Try picking from the rainbow of colours available to maximize variety. Eat non-starchy vegetables such as spinach, carrots, broccoli or green beans with meals

- Choose whole grain foods over processed grain products. Try brown rice with your stir fry or whole wheat spaghetti with your favourite pasta sauce

- Include dried beans (like kidney or pinto beans) and lentils into your meals

- Include fish in your meals 2–3 times a week

- Choose lean meats like cuts of beef and pork that end in "loin" such as pork loin and sirloin

- Remove the skin from chicken and turkey
- Choose non-fat dairy such as skimmed milk, non-fat yogurt and non-fat cheese
- Choose water and calorie-free "diet" drinks instead of regular soda, fruit punch, sweet tea and other sugar-sweetened drinks
- Choose liquid oils for cooking instead of solid fats that can be high in saturated and trans fats
- Remember that fats are high in calories. If you're trying to lose weight, watch your portion sizes of added fats
- Cut back on high-calorie snack foods and desserts like chips, cookies, cakes and full-fat ice cream
- Eating too much of even healthful foods can lead to weight gain. Watch your portion sizes

Patient.co.uk

The website www.patient.co.uk provides information both for patients and professionals on all sorts of health topics. Advantages of this resource are firstly its availability – it is linked to a major UK clinical software system in primary care, and secondly that it provides the same advice to both patients and clinicians but at two different levels. Patient UK articles and leaflets give a 'plain English' version, whilst 'Patient Plus' resources cover the issues in more depth. Both are available for patients as well as their professionals. All of the materials can be printed off during consultations or in the patient's home.

Summary

People living with diabetes have an increasing need to access support from local, national and global organisations offering practical advice, help and advocacy. Clinicians need to be able to signpost such people towards the most valuable resources in order to maximise their benefits. Patient groups have an important role in funding diabetes research and in advising professional and governmental policy makers. They are an extremely active force in the battle to defeat diabetes.

Further reading

Jaiveer P, Saraswathy J, Lee JD, Morrissey J, Patel V. The Alphabet Strategy – A tool to achieve clinical trials standards in routine practice? *Br J Diabetes Vasc Dis* 2003;**3**:410–3.
American Diabetes Association www.diabetes.org
Diabetes UK www.diabetes.org.uk
International Diabetes Federation www.idf.org
Patient.co.uk www.patient.co.uk

Index

Note: page numbers in *italics* refer to figures and boxes; Page numbers in **bold** refer to tables